The Weight Loss Revolution

The Weight Loss Revolution

Weight Loss Drugs and
How to Use Them

Dr Ambrish Mithal
with
Shivam Vij

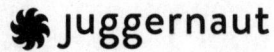

JUGGERNAUT BOOKS
C-I-128, First Floor, Sangam Vihar, Near Holi Chowk,
New Delhi 110080, India

First published by Juggernaut Books 2025

Copyright © Ambrish Mithal 2025

10 9 8 7 6 5 4 3 2 1

P-ISBN: 9789353456979
E-ISBN: 9789353453039

The views and opinions expressed in this book are the author's own.
The facts contained herein were reported to be true as on the date
of publication by the author to the publishers of the book, and the
publishers are not in any way liable for their accuracy or veracity.

All rights reserved. No part of this publication may be reproduced,
transmitted, or stored in a retrieval system in any form or by any
means without the written permission of the publisher.

Typeset in Adobe Caslon Pro by R. Ajith Kumar, Noida

Printed at Thomson Press India Ltd

To the brave souls who've survived countless diet plans

Contents

Introduction   1

1. It Started with a Lizard   11
2. Who Should Take Them, Who Should Not   28
3. Side Effects and How to Manage Them   46
4. The GLP-1 Journey   75
5. The ABCD of Weight Gain   94
6. The Chakravyuh: Why It's So Hard to Lose Weight   112
7. The Happy Side Effects   136
8. A Revolution in Diabetes Management   152
9. The GLP-1 Decade Has Only Just Begun   172

Bibliography   188
Acknowledgements   199
A Note on the Authors   200

Introduction

Obesity is a word that conjures up all kinds of thoughts and images, from the corpulent uncle who is the butt of family jokes, to Santa Claus ho-ho-ho-ing his way to our homes on Christmas, to the comedian Hardy of *Laurel and Hardy* fame. All of these are seemingly happy, jolly people. Scratch the surface, however, and you will often find an unhappy person longing to be thin.

How we perceive 'fatness' or obesity depends on prevailing social norms. In essence, **obesity means the presence of excess body fat that can impair health.** The word 'obesity' is derived from the French *obésité*, which comes from the Latin *obesitas*, which means 'fatness', and *obesus*, which means 'something that's eaten itself fat'. The roots are '*ob*', which means 'over', and '*edere*', which means 'to eat'.

Obesity has existed for thousands of years, but it was rare in ancient times. A famous 25,000-year-old sculpture, the Venus of Willendorf, housed in Vienna, shows the torso of a morbidly obese woman. The ancient Greek physician Hippocrates mentioned that sudden death was more common in those who were fat rather than lean. Other Greek physicians noted the association of obesity with infertility and irregular menses. Ancient Indian physicians Charaka and Sushruta astutely observed the tendency of sedentary, overweight individuals to develop diabetes and proposed exercise as a solution. (Wherever we say diabetes in this book, we mean type 2, unless otherwise mentioned.)

In the Middle Ages, food was scarce, and obesity was a status symbol of wealth and health. Throughout most of the nineteenth century, carrying an extra 10–20 kg of fat was considered healthy, with the hope that it would help a person cope with an extended illness. Being thin was not considered healthy and attributed to anxiety or disease. Instead of reducing caloric intake, the emphasis was on how to gain weight.

Only in the latter half of the nineteenth century did being fat begin to be regarded as aesthetically unpleasant. Its association with increased mortality was recognized only in the twentieth century. In other words, before it was realized that fat was bad for health, it was considered ugly. This continues to be the case in society today.

In his 1892 textbook *The Principles and Practice of Medicine*, the legendary Sir William Osler attributed obesity to 'overeating, a *vice* which is more prevalent and only a little behind overdrinking in its disastrous effects'.

Introduction

In recent decades, obesity has become a global epidemic due to shifts in food consumption patterns and is recognized as a chronic disease with numerous adverse health consequences.

While the current understanding of obesity as a disease is accepted by much of the medical fraternity, it is still regarded as a predominantly cosmetic problem by the general community. It surprises me that many of my patients don't realize the association between obesity and diabetes or heart disease. Patients often ask me how they can 'reverse' or get rid of their diabetes. When I tell them that the way to get rid of diabetes is to lose weight, most find it hard to believe. That, for me, is one of the biggest challenges in managing obesity: making people understand that obesity is a health problem and the reason for their diabetes, breathlessness, knee pain, high blood pressure, high bad cholesterol, and so on. Another challenge is explaining that integral to their treatment is lifestyle modification, which is daunting for most and impossible for many.

Over the years, the problem with clinically managing obesity has been the lack of tools. The history of anti-obesity drugs is full of failures. None of the anti-obesity medicines developed before semaglutide and tirzepatide (Ozempic and Mounjaro) have stood the test of time. The older drugs were either not effective enough, or their side effects were unacceptable. These new drugs are based on glucagon-like peptide-1 (GLP-1), a natural hormone produced in the body in response to food. The drugs mimic the hormone.

Until recently, the only option for the severely obese patient was bariatric surgery. The procedure entails making the stomach smaller or bypassing it altogether. While the benefits of bariatric surgery are well documented and proven, most of my patients do not agree to undergo it for fear of side effects or just the fear of surgery per se.

The extent of weight loss that can be achieved by surgery far exceeds that of any other method – sometimes to the tune of 40–50 kg. I have been a strong advocate of bariatric surgery for appropriately selected patients: those with a body mass index (BMI) over 40 (in some cases, with a BMI over 35). Unfortunately, many patients regain weight even after losing it through bariatric surgery. This happens because the stomach pouch expands again. After bariatric surgery, some patients think they no longer have to care about diet and exercise. That is not the case. If your doctor has told you to drink a lot of fluids after a bariatric surgery, it can't be sugar soda.

Our understanding of how obesity develops has also been limited. We have not been able to move beyond the fundamental axiom that it reflects the imbalance between what goes in (energy consumed through food) and what comes out (energy spent through physical activity). We haven't made much progress in understanding why, with apparently similar diets, one individual puts on weight while the other does not. Or, when two friends join a slimming programme, why one loses 10 kg, while the other struggles to lose even 2 kg. Or, why some of our 'foodie' friends think and dream about food all the time and cannot curtail their food cravings. It has been said that the decision to lose weight has to be made by the brain, not by the stomach. It is now understood that this may have something to do with the way the brain is wired and how the hormone–brain axis works differently for some people. The success of GLP-1 drugs is helping us understand these mechanisms better.

Before the modern crop of GLP-1 drugs was discovered, we had no way to address this brain defect. **Currently available GLP-1 drugs produce weight loss between 10 and 20 per cent of total body weight, which is immensely beneficial for health. Future drugs from the same stable may cause even greater weight loss.** These drugs fill a huge void that existed in the field of obesity management.

These days, I often get patients who have regained weight after bariatric surgery and now want GLP-1 drugs. There is no harm in using GLP-1 drugs for such patients. A patient who needs to lose 60 kg may first lose some of it through GLP-1 drugs, and the rest through bariatric surgery. This shall also make the surgery easier. A big advantage of GLP-1 drugs over bariatric surgery is the greater surety that the lost weight won't return *until the drug is continued*.

The best way to tackle obesity is to prevent it from developing in the first place. This can only be done by a judicious combination of a healthy diet, regular exercise, adequate sleep and low stress. In India, about half of the population is overweight or obese, despite a high simultaneous prevalence of malnutrition – a double whammy. As economic growth continues, food becomes more abundant, and fast or junk food permeates every nook and corner of India; obesity rates can only rocket skywards.

A study published in *The Lancet* estimates that a third of India's population will be overweight or obese by 2050. So much so that, in February of 2025, Prime Minister Narendra Modi highlighted the issue of rising obesity in India and suggested that people reduce their consumption of edible oil.

The cost of unhealthy 'junk' food is always lower than healthy food. Sweetened beverages cost less than milk; candy costs less than fruits. This drives people further towards unhealthy choices. To expect that medication can be a major method to combat the *public health* problem of obesity and diabetes in India is unrealistic. What these drugs do is provide a *medical* means to treat the disease, something that did not exist so far. They can provide relief to millions who are suffering the ill effects of obesity and prevent many from developing them.

When a drug captures the imagination of the public, like GLP-1 drugs definitely have, it moves from medical conferences to daily news headlines, with everyone forming their own opinion. Misinformation and half-baked information abound in the media. I have not read so much about any medical issue, other than Covid-19, in the media. Social media takes this to another level. There are some who believe that GLP-1 drugs are the panacea for all chronic diseases and that everybody should be taking them. Then there are others who feel that they should not be taken by anyone, even those suffering from obesity and its comorbidities. They say these drugs are very 'new', we do not have enough experience and they have not been studied well enough yet. Some others are terrified of side effects, both known and unknown.

The exaggeration of side effects is a big challenge. There is a risk of side effects with every medication we use. To say that a drug *can* have side effects is very different from saying that it *will*. This is true of most decisions in life. When we buy a new car, we check all the safety measures, yet it does not guarantee that we will not have an accident. We need to know how common a side effect is, and which patients are more likely to experience it.

Using any drug is always a benefit versus risk calculation. We forget that a commonly used non-prescription drug like aspirin can cause bleeding, which can even be fatal. Even low-dose aspirin, used commonly to reduce the risk of heart attacks, can cause brain haemorrhages in two out of every 1,000 people who take it. It is a known hazard, and it doesn't make newspaper headlines. The benefits of aspirin far outweigh the risks for people who have had a heart attack or are at high risk of getting one. Yet, the risks may exceed the benefits in those who are over seventy-five or are healthy. All individuals are not the same.

Choosing the right candidate, the right dose and appropriate medical supervision are essential. This will ensure maximal efficacy and minimize the risk of adverse effects. I am of the belief that we should repose our faith in our doctor. Yes, we should ask them all about side effects before embarking on a new treatment, but ultimately, it is the doctor who will have the knowledge, experience and perspective to guide you.

This book is meant to help the general public understand GLP-1 drugs from the right perspective, drawing on the latest research and clinical outcomes. It is not intended as individual medical advice.

With GLP-1 drugs, minor side effects are common and manageable, but major side effects are exceedingly rare. Those who worry excessively about the side effects need to keep in mind the risks of obesity and uncontrolled diabetes, which are powerfully and consistently reduced by these drugs. Novel and sometimes unexpected benefits of GLP-1 drugs are being reported every day. It is, however, important for physicians to keep their antennae up and report all minor and major side effects. This process, known as pharmacovigilance, is a public health responsibility.

Undoubtedly, GLP-1 medications are the biggest drug discovery in recent times. They could considerably improve the prevention and management of several non-communicable diseases. Their discovery has unlocked new pathways and approaches to tackle disease. The ability of some newer GLP-1 drugs to act via additional pathways, like glucose-dependent insulinotropic polypeptide (GIP) and glucagon, opens up exciting possibilities. In the future, we may see greater efficacy, specific organ-targeted effects, reduction of unpleasant side effects and easier oral administration schedules. The speed of research in this field is astounding. New drugs are expected almost every year for the next few years. We are living in the GLP-1 decade!

One of the biggest challenges to the widespread adoption of GLP-1 medications is their high cost, which puts them out of reach for most, especially in India. The success of these drugs has significantly impacted the economy of the countries where they originated – Denmark and the USA. The good news is that the cost is expected to decline significantly when new molecules emerge and the patents on some of the earlier ones, like semaglutide, expire. I expect that in 2026, the price of GLP-1 drugs will crash in India.

Another issue with these drugs has been a shortage of supplies. The innovator companies were possibly caught off guard by the enormous demand for these drugs, and there was a global shortage for an extended period of time. I understand that it has been largely resolved. Going off-patent will allow generic manufacturers to enter the fray, and I hope drug shortages will be a thing of the past.

In this book, I will try to answer many of the questions that have been bothering you. Many friends are taking these drugs, should I try them too? Can I use them to lose just 2 kg for my daughter's wedding so that I can fit into my old dress again? Am I putting myself at risk by using these new drugs to control my diabetes? Will they damage my organs? The questions that I get asked in the clinic and on the phone on a daily basis are all answered here.

1

It Started with a Lizard

I remember giving talks in the early 2000s about the dream of every endocrinologist: an anti-diabetes drug that would control blood sugar without lowering it below normal levels and cause weight loss instead of weight gain.

For persons with type 2 diabetes, medicines are needed to bring down their blood sugar levels, but the drugs can sometimes cause them to plummet, a condition called hypoglycaemia. Symptoms of hypoglycaemia include trembling, sweating, sudden hunger, fatigue, anxiety, confusion, dizziness and irritability. If not addressed immediately with food, it can be dangerous.

Some diabetes drugs cause weight gain. The increasing weight worsens the diabetes, requiring more medication. This becomes a vicious cycle.

The dream of having a drug that caused weight loss and no hypoglycaemia came true one day. That day wasn't when

Ozempic was approved for treating diabetes. It was not the first 'weight-loss' drug, and it is not the last. No doubt very effective, it has the distinction of becoming a household name, a by-word for all such medications we call GLP-1 drugs. However, the first such drug was approved in 2005. It was called exenatide, sold under the brand name Byetta.

The story begins with a lizard. This is no ordinary lizard. It is one of a few lizard varieties that are venomous. It can be up to two feet long and weigh about 2 kg. Found mostly in south-western United States (US), it is a slow-moving, colourful desert reptile that spends most of its time hidden in burrows. This lizard eats often only in spring, and can eat meals as large as one-third of its body weight. Then it stores fat in its tail and doesn't need to eat for months. It is called the Gila monster.

In the 1970s, Dr John Eng was studying the venom of the Gila monster. He found that it had a peptide (chain of amino acids) called exendin-4, which was similar to the hormone GLP-1 found in human intestines. Both hormones were produced in response to food and helped release insulin, but the difference was that the Gila monster's exendin-4 lasted much longer in the blood than the human GLP-1.

All of us produce GLP-1 as a response to eating food, but it disappears in no time. It has a 'half-life' of just two minutes, meaning that half of GLP-1 produced in our bodies in response to food is degraded within two minutes. This is because of an enzyme found throughout the human body called DPP-4, which breaks down GLP-1.

The earliest trials gave a continuous infusion of GLP-1 to test if and how it was affecting sugar levels and appetite. That, obviously, was not practically feasible. Hence, the challenge in making a GLP-1-like drug was to prolong its action in the body.

If scientists could use what they learnt from the Gila monster's venomous saliva to create a drug that could stay longer than the natural GLP-1 in the human body, they could make the pancreas of patients with diabetes produce more natural insulin, which would manage their blood sugar levels without increasing weight.

In 1987, Amylin Pharmaceuticals and Eli Lilly and Company teamed up to try and make such a drug possible. After years of research and development, they came up with exenatide – a synthetic version of exendin-4, the peptide found in the Gila monster. It was only in 2005 that exenatide was approved for public use by the US Food and Drug Administration (US FDA), and sold under the brand name Byetta, becoming the first GLP-1 drug. By 2007, I was prescribing it to my patients in India.

Exenatide enhances natural insulin production only when blood sugar is high, thus removing the risk of hypoglycaemia. It suppresses glucagon, a hormone that raises blood sugar. It slows gastric emptying, making food move slowly in the stomach and thus letting the patient feel full for longer. It also reduces appetite, thus helping with weight loss. It has to be injected subcutaneously (under the skin) twice a day, an hour before breakfast and dinner each.

Over the years, my colleagues and I have published many research papers on GLP-1 drugs by measuring their impact on our patients in India. In a paper published in 2013, we observed that our patients with diabetes lost 4–5 kg weight after taking exenatide (Byetta) for six months. It also helped in sugar control. However, Byetta's gastrointestinal side effects like nausea and vomiting were quite harsh, and it had to be injected twice a day, limiting its adoption.

Sadly, the Gila monster is at risk of extinction, affected by climate change and drought.

While Byetta was a product of learning from its venom, scientists were also working on a parallel track to make a drug that would entirely mimic the human GLP-1 and stay longer in the bloodstream.

Five years later, in 2010, came liraglutide, first sold under the brand name Victoza, which had to be injected only once a day. This was an important landmark since it was the first GLP-1 drug to be entirely based on the human hormone. It produced good results in controlling sugar levels. In 2015, liraglutide became the first GLP-1 drug in the US to be approved specifically for obesity, under the brand name Saxenda. Some were able to lose 8–10 per cent of their total body weight with this drug.

In 2014, there was albiglutide (Tanzeum), followed by dulaglutide (Trulicity). Trulicity had to be taken only once a week, marking a major advance in enhancing the convenience of GLP-1 treatment. This was possible because scientists figured out how to make the drug last longer in the bloodstream, extending its half-life. The drug rapidly gained widespread popularity because of its ease of use. Meanwhile, scientists had also succeeded in making a long-acting (weekly) version of Byetta.

Most of these older drugs are still in use because they either serve a specific purpose for patients with diabetes, such as when combined with insulin in the same injection pen, or are cheap and easily available now that their patents have expired.

In December 2017 came semaglutide, sold under the brand name Ozempic. This was a major turning point since it demonstrated an average weight loss of 15 per cent of total body weight for patients, and up to 20 per cent in some lucky ones.

Converting the injectable drug into an oral pill was not easy. In 2019, Novo Nordisk got approval for semaglutide in pill form, under the brand name Rybelsus. This is the first and – so far – only GLP-1 pill. It has been approved and available in India since 2022.

In 2022, tirzepatide was approved by the US FDA under the brand name Mounjaro. It was launched in India in March 2025. Tirzepatide mimics the action of not one but two hormones: GLP-1 and GIP. Patients can lose up to 22.5 per cent of their total body weight with this drug.

To understand the world of weight-loss drugs, it is important to appreciate this history. It has been twenty years now since the first one, Byetta, hit the market.

The Discovery of GLP-1

Hormones are messengers in the body, carrying a specific message to the brain and other organs. Most people reading this book would have heard of some of the well-known hormones such as testosterone, oestrogen, cortisol, insulin and melatonin. There are a large number of hormones in the human body, and many more are still being discovered. When I was a postgraduate student of endocrinology at the All India Institute of Medical Sciences (AIIMS) in Delhi in the 1980s, it used to take a month for a hormone blood test to come in, if at all. Today, patients are angsty if they don't get it the same day. The study of hormones is called endocrinology. A doctor trained in endocrinology is an endocrinologist.

It Started with a Lizard

In 1964, scientists researching diabetes found something counterintuitive: glucose given orally raised insulin levels in the human body more than glucose given intravenously. This meant that something in the stomach makes the pancreas produce more insulin and helps break down food. They concluded that there are some hormones found in the gut that increase insulin levels. It was not known what these hormones were or how many in number. They were named incretin hormones – incretin means intestinal hormones that increase insulin secretion.

The first incretin hormone to be identified was GIP by John E. Brown in 1970. However, it was not found to be very effective when used as a drug for diabetes. GIP initially stood for gastric inhibitory polypeptide but was later renamed glucose-dependent insulinotropic polypeptide.

I was in training as an endocrinologist, when, in 1986, the discovery of GLP-1 was announced. It was found to be a key hormone responsible for regulating blood sugar in humans. I remember participating in a departmental discussion on the findings in the journal club. The importance of this new discovery was hotly debated.

The discovery took place at the Massachusetts General Hospital in Boston. Yugoslavia-born Svetlana Mojsov, a molecular biologist, began to delve into the mysteries of GLP-1 after looking at glucagon, the sugar-raising hormone. In a different lab in the same research hospital, endocrinologist Dr Joel Francis Habener and his team had also been looking at glucagon and found a stretch of amino acids that resembled glucagon but was different. Due to the structural similarity, they named it glucagon-like peptide-1 or GLP-1.

Mojsov hypothesized that a particular string of amino acids, 7-31, was GLP-1. She then began to test if it was present in the intestines as suspected. Until then, there was only one known incretin, GIP, and it had failed to stimulate much insulin in trials. Mojsov isolated GLP-1 in glass vials and injected its antibodies into a rabbit to test the response.

Dr Habener began to study the biology of GLP-1 with a new colleague, Dr Daniel J. Drucker. They approached Dr Mojsov to collaborate on GLP-1. Soon, the trio was able to establish its presence in rat intestines in a landmark paper. Then they went for the next step, looking to see if increasing GLP-1 levels corresponded with increase in insulin. 'It was a beautiful experiment,' she would later say about how the rat pancreas responded with a proportionate increase in insulin to the GLP-1 injections. The team then went on to successfully do the experiment in humans.

It often happens in science that two different teams make the same discovery or invention around the same time in different research laboratories. Dr Jens Juul Holst and his team in Copenhagen published the same research on

GLP-1 and its insulin-stimulating powers roughly during the same period (mid-1980s) as did the trio in Boston.

However, the patents were registered solely in Dr Habener's name. As GLP-1 drugs took off, the fame and patent royalties excluded Dr Svetlana Mojsov, who had to hire lawyers to have her name included in the patents.

Dr Daniel Drucker now works as an obesity researcher at the Lunenfeld-Tanenbaum Research Institute, Mount Sinai Hospital, in Toronto. Forty years after he was part of the team that identified and named GLP-1, he continues to research GLP-1 drugs, conduct experiments and publish findings. He is today the most influential scientist in the field.

How GLP-1 Works

After we eat food, GLP-1 tells the pancreas to produce insulin. Insulin lowers blood sugar. Simultaneously, GLP-1 reduces the release of glucagon, a hormone that increases blood sugar. GLP-1 also delays how quickly food leaves the stomach, making you feel full. It also tells the brain to reduce appetite. Thus, GLP-1 is a key spoke in the wheel of metabolism.

GLP-1 'receptors' are found all over the body, including in the brain, heart, gut, small intestine, liver, pancreas, kidneys, lungs and even in the blood vessels and fat tissues.

Think of these receptors as switches. The pathway of the drug begins with reaching the switches and turning them on, which activates a chain of reactions and processes, leading to biological effects.

GLP-1 drugs are 'agonists', synthetically produced molecules that mimic the natural hormone, travelling to GLP-1 receptors and activating them. GLP-1, both the hormone and the drugs that mimic it, stabilizes blood sugar and reduces weight through four actions: by making the person feel full for longer; by making the pancreas produce more natural insulin but only in response to high blood sugar; by reducing the sugar-raising hormone glucagon; and by telling the brain to make the person eat less. This quadruple action produces remarkable results and makes these drugs ideal for people with or without diabetes who have excessive body fat.

It is important to appreciate here that GLP-1 lowers blood sugar only within the normal range, never below it, and only in response to high sugar levels. This glucose-dependent insulin stimulation ensures that the patient is not at risk of hypoglycaemia.

GLP-1 has a sibling, GIP, which mainly helps boost insulin release and does not have any effect on stomach emptying. Scientists found that GIP alone was not producing significant results in trials, and it seemed that GLP-1 was the hormone to target.

What if we targeted both GLP-1 and GIP? Not many scientists shared the hope that adding GIP agonists to GLP-1 would lead to better results. German scientist Matthias Tschöp and his colleagues persisted with the idea that doing so would lead to better results. They were eventually proved right, and that is how we got tirzepatide (Mounjaro), which produces greater weight loss than other GLP-1 drugs.

Patients taking GLP-1 drugs often find they don't feel like eating – their appetite is reduced – and don't think about food all day like they used to. They also find that they feel full very quickly once they start eating – improvement in satiety. Many say that they are now more inclined to eat healthier foods, and some complain they no longer find eating pleasurable. All of this seems to suggest that GLP-1 drugs are acting powerfully on the brain, apart from slowing gastric emptying and stimulating insulin.

It is their actions on the brain that make semaglutide (Ozempic) and tirzepatide (Mounjaro) path-breaking. This has opened up a world of possibilities that is being explored in trials. They could even play a role in alleviating Parkinson's and Alzheimer's disease.

A growing number of trials are showing us that GLP-1 and GIP hormones are beneficial for much more than metabolism. There is increasing evidence that they improve cardiovascular health and reduce the risk of heart attacks and brain stroke. Many patients taking these drugs say that their desire to drink alcohol has gone down significantly, which is leading to research on the use of GLP-1s for addiction treatment. Large trials are underway to study if they can help wean people off smoking and drugs.

The beneficial effects of GLP-1 drugs on kidney health and fatty liver have now been seen across the world. They have already been approved in the US for some conditions, especially for patients of obesity and diabetes, including sleep apnoea, heart disease and chronic kidney disease. Many of these benefits are, of course, a direct result of weight loss. But there may be more to it. They work directly on the brain and possibly on other organs as well.

A Holistic Approach

When I started as an endocrinologist forty years ago, there were only three tools to address diabetes: insulin, metformin and sulphonylureas. All three were focused on controlling blood sugar. It may surprise you that the concept of tight glucose control with intensive treatment was not established at that time.

In the mid-1990s, a landmark study called the UKPDS, or United Kingdom Prospective Diabetes Study, demonstrated that good glucose control resulted in reduced diabetes complications. The focus moved to better control.

I remember saying often in my talks in the early 2000s that the only thing that matters is controlling blood sugar. How you do it does not matter. That is no longer true.

Today, we have been able to move beyond mere glucose management. With newer drugs like GLP-1 receptor agonists and SGLT2 inhibitors (which throw out excess glucose through urine) we are able to address underlying issues, such as obesity and metabolic health, and thus look at diabetes holistically. These molecules also reduce the risk of long-term complications, such as those involving the heart, kidneys and liver, independent of their actions on blood glucose.

Let's take the example of a patient I saw recently. He was fifty years old, on forty units of insulin a day along with oral medication, yet his HbA1c, a measure of average blood sugar levels in the last two–three months, was 8.5 per cent (the target is to keep it under 7 per cent). He was obese, weighing 90 kg, and his BMI was 31. I prescribed him Rybelsus, the oral form of semaglutide.

The first thing I noticed was the decline in his insulin dosage. I reduced the amount of prescribed insulin, and yet he continued to get attacks of hypoglycaemia (sugar levels below 70 mg/dL). The dosage of oral medications (sulphonylureas) was then reduced. As mentioned earlier, sulphonylureas are popular glucose-lowering drugs that can cause hypoglycaemia. His insulin dosage was halved in just four weeks. In three months, he was only on metformin and semaglutide. His HbA1c now is 6.5 per cent. He does not get hypoglycaemia any more, and so long as he continues to be on these two medications, there is no risk of it in the future too. The absence of hypoglycaemia means that better control is possible with less risk. Besides this, semaglutide reduces his risk of heart attacks, the progression of his kidney complications, and squeezes out fat from his liver. And he has lost 4 kg too! In other words, this patient is in a much better place now than three months ago.

We have now started prescribing GLP-1 drugs to patients early in the course of diabetes, helping them lose weight and thus increasing the possibility of inducing remission. Metformin is still the frontline drug given to people when they're first diagnosed with diabetes, but I foresee that changing in favour of GLP-1 drugs in the near future. I have many patients who do not need to take metformin any more – just a GLP-1 drug is enough to maintain both their sugar and weight.

Type 2 diabetes is only one of many diseases caused by the meta-disease of obesity. For people who are overweight or obese and are unable to lose weight through lifestyle modification, these drugs offer a way out.

For overweight and obese patients who have pre-diabetes or have other obesity-related health issues, GLP-1 drugs may be useful in not only preventing future diabetes but also reducing their weight. Excess body fat is the driver of most non-communicable diseases that can be prevented with weight loss.

Diabetes reduces the average lifespan by seven to ten years, and excessive body fat accelerates ageing. By making people healthier, GLP-1 drugs could add many years to their lives.

Takeaway

GLP-1 and GIP are natural hormones found in the body that help regulate hunger, satiety, stomach movement and insulin secretion. Drugs that mimic these hormones have been around since 2005. Ozempic and Mounjaro are only the latest drugs in the series. Since the action of natural GLP-1 lasts only a few minutes, the development of GLP-1 drugs has sought to extend the duration of action, and to preferentially enhance weight-loss properties.

PATIENT STORY

AKSHAT RATHEE, 44

Both sets of my grandparents had diabetes and hypertension, so there was always a genetic predisposition for diabetes. I gained weight with age, work stress and a lot of travel.

I was 101 kg. My HbA1c was a worrying 11. Dr Mithal had put me on a total of 11 medicines. I would often forget to take them or not take them when I was supposed to. My compliance rate with these medicines was about 40 per cent. Some of them were giving me terrible side effects. So I went back to Dr Mithal and said that this was not going to work. I travel twenty days a month and have a stressful work life. He asked me to try a GLP-1 drug. Now I take just two pills a day, a daily metformin along with a statin for cholesterol. My sugar and weight are both coming down with a weekly Mounjaro injection. My current weight is 88 kg. I am targeting 82 kg.

I started with Ozempic 0.25 mg and it had no effect on me – no side effects, no weight loss, no sugar control. I increased it to 0.5 mg, which had some impact on my sugar levels but no impact on my weight. Then came 1 mg, which was good for both sugar and weight. Ozempic

2 mg produced further weight loss but had no incremental impact on my blood sugar. It became difficult to get the 2 mg pen, so I switched to Mounjaro.

However, there was a month in between when I was on neither of them. In this one month alone, I gained back 5 kg of the 12 kg I had lost. I started with Mounjaro 2.5 mg, on which I gained another 1 kg weight in a month. The next dose was 5 mg, which gave me some weight loss but very slowly. Dr Mithal then made me jump straight to 10 mg, which has been perfect for me. I'm now losing 1 kg a week on 10 mg. My HbA1c is down to 6.1.

Ozempic made me gassy and irritable; it parched the sides of my tongue and I felt thirstier. With Mounjaro, I face a lot of burping and flatulence only for one day, the day after I take the injection.

From three heavy meals, I am down to eating two light meals, breakfast at 9.30 a.m. and dinner at 7 p.m., and nothing in between. From eating three parathas, I am in a situation where I can barely finish one. I have higher energy levels and my cholesterol levels have also improved.

I have friends who needed to lose weight, and I suggested they take one of these drugs. Some tried but gave up – they wanted the joy of eating three parathas. I want the joy of being healthy for my newborn child.

2

Who Should Take Them, Who Should Not

Whether or not you should take GLP-1 drugs is best determined by your doctor. A qualified endocrinologist needs to look at your medical history, pre-existing diseases and blood test reports to make the decision.

This warning is important because every patient is different, with different risk profiles and complications. This chapter is a general discussion on what kind of patients should be taking GLP-1 drugs and who should not be taking them. Note that these guidelines keep evolving with time as new studies come out and make us wiser. That is why it is all the more important to consult a doctor before starting on a serious long-term medicine like GLP-1. It is not an over-the-counter painkiller.

It is important to educate the public about GLP-1 drugs and their uses to ensure correct use and prevent misuse. Within the next two years, we are going to see an explosion of GLP-1 drugs in India. Given the hype around them, the public needs to understand who they are for.

Bull's Eye

The ideal candidate for GLP-1 drugs is someone who has type 2 diabetes, and is overweight or obese. The question is, how do we define overweight and obese?

Conventional definitions of these terms have been challenged. Endocrinologists have been questioning the use of BMI as the sole parameter of obesity for some time now.

Body mass index is a number derived by dividing a person's weight in kg, with the square of their height in metres (BMI = weight (kg) / height^2 (m^2)). Several easy BMI calculators are available online. It is a useful index but can often be misleading, especially among Indians. Many of us tend to have more abdominal and visceral fat, which is the most harmful fat, affecting our critical organs.

Someone with a high BMI may have a lot of muscle or bone mass. Someone with a moderately high or even normal-range BMI may have excessive body fat percentage, and worse, this body fat may be concentrated around the abdomen, where it is most harmful to the internal organs. Online BMI calculators also have the limitation of being made for the Western population. For Indians, the cut-offs are lower. BMI calculators you'll find online suggest that the cut-off for being overweight is BMI 25 and for obesity it is 30. However, since Indians develop metabolic complications at a lower BMI, the cut-offs for Indians as suggested by the Endocrine Society of India are 23 and 25. This is a revision of the earlier understanding that the Indian obesity cut-off should be 28.

For a clearer picture of overweight and obesity, it is useful to look at waist circumference, waist-to-hip ratio and body fat percentage.

To calculate the waist-to-hip ratio, first measure the waist circumference. This is done just above the belly button. Then measure the hip circumference. This is done at the widest point the measuring tape goes around the hips. Dividing the waist circumference with the hip circumference gives the waist-to-hip ratio.

The table below gives the acceptable upper limits on these counts for both South Asian and Western populations.

Table 1: Upper normal limits for South Asians and Western populations, measured through waist circumference, waist-to-hip ratio, and body fat percentage

Markers	Level in South Asians	Western Population
Waist circumference		
Men	≥90 cm	≥102 cm
Women	≥80 cm	≥88 cm
Waist-to-hip ratio		
Men	≥0.9	≥0.9
Women	≥0.8	≥0.8
Body fat percentage		
Men	≥20%	≥25%
Women	≥33%	≥35%

There is a lack of consensus on what the Indian body fat percentage cut off should be given the preponderance of central obesity. The Endocrine Society of India has suggested 25 per cent for men and 30 per cent for women.

A person with a BMI of 26 may not appear overweight but could have body fat as high as 38 per cent, concentrated around the belly. Body mass index works on the assumption that all fat is the same. Yet the fat around arms or thighs is not as harmful. Many Indians tend to be 'skinny fat', having thin arms and legs but a big belly.

Roughly speaking, 90 per cent of the fat in a person is what can be seen outwardly. This fat is subcutaneous or under the skin. The remaining 10 per cent is inside the abdomen, called visceral fat, as it surrounds the internal organs (viscera), such as the liver and kidneys. It is the fat you can't pinch.

Hence, there may be a diabetes patient who might not appear obese, may only be a little overweight, but might have very high visceral fat.

The ideal way to determine the degree of body fat is by estimating body composition using a magnetic resonance imaging (MRI) machine. This is rarely done in clinical practice. The DXA machine, which is commonly used to measure bone density, provides an accurate measure too. However, this requires an appointment and a separate visit. A quick method which can be used in the clinic and is fairly reliable is a body composition analyser using bioimpedance technology. One only has to stand on it for 2–3 minutes, and a report is generated giving body fat, muscle and bone mass figures for hands, abdomen and legs.

Abdominal circumference, or a waist-to-hip ratio, gives a fair estimate of visceral fat content. These are simple clinical measures that can be used in any clinic. A waist circumference of over 80 cm in women and over 90 cm in men is considered high. A waist-to-hip ratio is also a good indirect measure of our visceral fat.

It is visceral fat that we need to target in the clinic. Visceral (or central) fat produces toxins, the bad hormones that increase insulin resistance and suppress insulin secretion. This needs to be understood by patients who may not have a very high BMI, but high levels of visceral fat could nevertheless be doing them great harm. Such a person, if he or she has diabetes, could benefit greatly from GLP-1 drugs.

Not all patients with type 2 diabetes are the same. There are at least five different 'clusters', as we call them. One such group is people who are overweight or obese, have an unhealthy diet, do little exercise and are insulin resistant. Even though their pancreas produces some insulin, their tissues do not respond to it. Such patients are ideal candidates for GLP-1 drugs. These drugs reduce their appetite and improve satiety. This reduction in food intake, along with stimulation of insulin secretion, which occurs soon after initiating treatment with GLP-1 drugs, will ensure rapid control of diabetes. Besides, overall diabetes management will become progressively easier as people lose weight.

Then there are those who, along with diabetes, have developed heart disease, kidney disease or fatty liver, or are at high risk for these complications. The evidence about the beneficial effects of GLP-1 drugs in reducing the risk and progression of these complications is solid and unequivocal. In all such cases, it is a no-brainer that they would benefit from GLP-1 drugs.

I am fairly certain that we are soon going to see GLP-1 drugs being prescribed to most persons with type 2

diabetes, unless there are contraindications (those patients where the drug could potentially be harmful). Medical guidelines are moving in this direction, but the movement has been slow because of the poor availability, high price and relative novelty of the drugs. As the drugs become more widely available and affordable, we will see them become the frontline defence against diabetes.

What if there is someone with mild diabetes, with an HbA1c of around 7, and metformin alone brings it down to 6.5? He is only a little overweight, let's say BMI 27. Should such a patient be taking GLP-1 today? If he tells me he is concerned about his long-term outcomes, given how even the best-managed diabetes can worsen with time, I would prefer that he takes GLP-1 drugs, provided he can afford them. I would like to bring down his BMI and protect his organs as much as I can.

People with Diabetes Who Should Not Take GLP-1

There are some people with diabetes who should not be prescribed GLP-1 drugs. These are patients who, in medical terminology, are in 'active catabolism' – patients who are so sick that they have started losing their body fat and muscle due to very high blood sugar levels. Such patients require insulin, not GLP-1s.

Those who are frail and elderly should also avoid GLP-1 drugs due to the muscle loss that inevitably accompanies fat loss. There are some studies suggesting that GLP-1 drugs may be safe and beneficial even for the frail, but as of now, I am not convinced that this would be the best thing to do as it could potentially worsen their frailty. The loss of muscle mass that accompanies rapid weight loss may enhance insulin resistance. More importantly, the risk of falling and consequent fractures may increase. Hip fracture is one of the most devastating occurrences in the elderly, and a loss in muscle mass increases the risk of hip fracture. In my opinion, the risks in such cases outweigh the potential benefits of GLP-1 drugs.

There is another cluster of type 2 diabetes where insulin deficiency is the dominant defect rather than insulin resistance. Such patients are often lean, and although they may have some resistance to insulin action, their primary issue is deficiency of insulin. Such patients rapidly lose response to oral anti-diabetic drugs and have to start taking insulin shots to manage their diabetes. GLP-1 drugs can help in controlling it too because of the insulin-stimulating action on the pancreas as well as reduction in food intake, but will probably not be as effective as they are for the insulin-resistant variety of diabetes. Unwanted weight loss may result in frailty and weakness in such patients. Such patients are, therefore, not ideal candidates for GLP-1.

GLP-1 drugs are not suitable for underweight type 2 diabetes patients, whose BMI is below 20, regardless of their age.

Type 1 diabetes patients should not take GLP-1 drugs except as an add-on to insulin. People with type 1 diabetes do not produce natural insulin, and the only medical redress is for them to take insulin shots. We usually think of type 1 diabetes patients as people who are thin. With the help of insulin shots, some people with type 1 diabetes also take to overeating and under-exercising, thus becoming overweight. Such type 1 diabetes patients would benefit from GLP-1 drugs. People with type 1 diabetes have to be careful when taking GLP-1 drugs – they cannot be the first option for them. If a type 1 diabetes patient is not overweight, GLP-1 drugs are not recommended.

People Without Diabetes Who Should Take GLP-1

Semaglutide was approved as a weight-loss drug in the US under the brand name Wegovy in 2021. Tirzepatide was similarly approved for weight loss under the brand name Zepbound in 2023. However, outside the US, Mounjaro is the brand name of tirzepatide for both diabetes and weight loss.

Rybelsus (oral semaglutide) was approved for diabetes in 2022 in India. Many endocrinologists, including me, have been prescribing it 'off-label' for weight loss in patients who may not have diabetes but nevertheless suffer from or are at great risk of obesity-related complications.

Tirzepatide, under the brand name Mounjaro, was approved by Indian drug regulators for both diabetes and 'chronic weight management' in India in September 2024 and made available in pharmacies in March 2025.

The US FDA has approved GLP-1 drugs for anyone with BMI above 30 and above. They have also approved them for anyone with BMI above 27 and above if they have any weight-related disease, such as diabetes, hypertension, fatty liver, sleep apnoea, osteoarthritis, and so on.

Indians often start experiencing such metabolic conditions when their BMI is around 25, which is why in the clinic we need to do body composition analysis more often and not go by BMI alone. This is particularly the case with people in the range of 23 to 27 BMI, where body fat percentage becomes critical in deciding whether medical intervention is required. It is possible that someone with a BMI of 26 has a high muscle mass and may, therefore, not need to worry about body fat.

GLP-1 drugs, including semaglutide, are also approved for children with obesity (above the age of twelve) or type 2 diabetes (above the age of ten) and are being increasingly used for them. However, concerns regarding nutritional imbalance as a result of marked reductions in food intake during the active growth period have been voiced.

Medical Conditions That Don't Let You Take GLP-1 Drugs

Pregnancy and Lactation

GLP-1 drugs are not approved for use during pregnancy and lactation. However, exposure to GLP-1 drugs in the first trimester was not associated with a risk of major birth defects when compared with diabetes or to overweight/obese women. Although limited by a small sample size, this study offers reassurance in cases of inadvertent exposure to GLP-1-RA during the first trimester of pregnancy.

Family History of Medullary Thyroid Cancer

Those who have a family history of medullary thyroid cancer, a rare variety of thyroid cancer, should not take GLP-1 drugs. This includes those with multiple endocrine neoplasia (MEN) syndrome. While an increased risk of developing medullary thyroid cancer with GLP-1 drugs has been shown in rats, human studies have yielded unconvincing and conflicting results. However, doctors and patients have to be mindful of this risk and measure serum calcitonin levels at the slightest suspicion. The common varieties of thyroid cancers have not been linked to GLP-1 drugs. Those who have or have had hypo- or hyperthyroidism can use GLP-1 drugs, if medically needed, without any concern. I recommend that all my patients on GLP-1 drugs check a serum calcitonin every three to six months. I also make it a point to physically examine the thyroid gland for any lumps or nodules.

History of Pancreatitis

If a patient has had pancreatitis in the past, they are not to be prescribed GLP-1 drugs. Pancreatitis is inflammation of the pancreas that overweight and diabetes patients are anyway more prone to; it is a painful and potentially dangerous condition. It usually causes acute abdominal pain. Recent data, however, points to the safety of GLP-1 medication in people who have a history of pancreatitis. This is true, in particular, for those who had a definite cause of pancreatitis, which has been corrected. A typical example would be gallstones causing pancreatitis. If the gall bladder has been surgically removed and the cause of pancreatitis is not there any more, studies suggest that GLP-1 drugs are safe for such patients. Even in the rare cases where a few have had pancreatitis after taking GLP-1 drugs, it is not clearly established if the medication was directly the cause of pancreatitis. Future trials and studies will help us better understand the relationship between GLP-1 drugs and pancreatitis. I have so far not had any patient who has suffered pancreatitis with the use of GLP-1.

It's also good to remember that a very popular and widely used group of oral drugs, aligned but not similar to GLP-1s, called DPP-4 inhibitors (sitagliptin, vildagliptin, linagliptin), has also been associated with pancreatitis. The number of prescriptions for DPP-4i is over ten fold of GLP-1 drugs. There, too, the jury is still out about the risk of pancreatitis.

One point that we always have to keep in mind is that obesity and diabetes patients are anyway at higher risk of pancreatitis. A recent study from the US showed that the risk of pancreatitis might actually be lower in those on GLP-1 because of improvement in both weight and diabetes control.

Active Proliferative Diabetic Retinopathy

Diabetes patients who have active proliferative retinopathy should not take GLP-1. It is an advanced stage of a condition that causes vision loss due to prolonged levels of high blood sugar. GLP-1 drugs have been found to worsen this condition in some patients. This is most likely due to a sudden drop in sugar levels. This is known to be the case with insulin as well. Diabetes patients who take insulin and have diabetic retinopathy sometimes experience a similar aggravation of the eye condition when their sugar levels fall with insulin shots. The effect is likely temporary, but nonetheless, GLP-1 drugs are best avoided by such patients at present. Future studies will hopefully give us a better idea about whether and how this risk is manageable. My personal feeling is that these drugs will be used for retinopathy patients in the future.

Prone to Nausea

Patients who are already prone to nausea and vomiting should not take GLP-1 medication. Many experience gastric side effects initially, but those who already have gastrointestinal issues may not be able to overcome the initial side effects. It must be said here that obese and overweight people often have heartburn and acid reflux due to gastroesophageal reflux disease (GERD). With GLP-1-induced weight loss, their GERD may only improve with time.

Sarcopenic Obesity

Indians, particularly the elderly, sometimes tend to have sarcopenic obesity – high fat with very low muscle mass along with poor bone density. In such cases, whether or not

GLP-1 drugs should be prescribed is a tricky decision the doctor has to make. Such patients should carefully follow their doctor's advice.

Cosmetic Considerations

Every now and then I get perfectly healthy people coming to me and asking for a GLP-1 prescription just to lose a few kilos solely for cosmetic considerations.

If GLP-1 drugs are safe for someone with BMI 30, why can't someone with BMI 24 not take it just to get a flat stomach and feel good about themselves?

A GLP-1 drug is a long-term medicine that should be taken only when lifestyle modification fails, and a person suffers from obesity-related problems, which may or may not include diabetes. Losing a few kilos is generally possible with lifestyle modifications. Ageing and physiology may make it difficult, yes, but lifestyle measures continue to be the mainstay of all obesity management. Using these medicines as a crutch without attempting lifestyle modification is not advisable.

While GLP-1s are safe for most people, there is no medication with zero risk. The next chapter will discuss side effects (and how to manage them), but the risk of even the rarest side effects is not worth taking for someone who has no medical reason to take it.

I had a fifty-year-old woman visit me in the clinic asking me for a prescription. She worked out regularly, weighed only 45 kg, and had a BMI of less than 19. In medical terms, she is underweight. She said she wanted to lose 3 kg.

'But Ma'am, why do you want to be 42 kg?' I asked.

'Because that was my weight when I was in college,' she said.

'But Ma'am you are no longer in college,' I replied.

I refused to give her a prescription. She came again to argue her case, and I had to disappoint her again. Cosmetic considerations alone are not an endocrinologist's remit. Even the slightest risk of side effects has to be justified in the clinic by medical need.

The desire to be so thin as to be medically underweight is also a behavioural disorder that won't result in the best health outcomes.

I get patients who have already procured Ozempic or Mounjaro injections from abroad, and they are lying in their refrigerators. They want me to say it is okay for them to take it. But when there is no medical need for them to do so, I can't take responsibility for any side effects they may get.

Takeaway

People who have obesity-related complications, such as diabetes, hypertension, heart disease, kidney disease, fatty liver, sleep apnoea, joint pain or polycystic ovary syndrome (PCOS), to name a few, are the ideal candidates to take GLP-1 drugs. People who are only a little overweight should continue to attempt to manage their weight with lifestyle modifications. The frail elderly, pregnant and lactating women, and those with a history of pancreatitis, gastroparesis, or advanced diabetic retinopathy should not use them. Let a doctor decide whether your particular health conditions make GLP-1 drugs necessary, safe and suitable for you.

> **PATIENT STORY**
>
> ---
>
> **NIKHIL SHARMA, 49***
>
> *I had been in the pre-diabetes range for years. My HbA1C used to be around 6. One day, it came out to be 7 in a test. Dr Mithal put me on metformin, but later he asked me to stop metformin and take Rybelsus instead. He also put me on dapagliflozin, an SGLT2 inhibitor that flushes out excess glucose through the urine.*
>
> *I started with Rybelsus 3 mg, increasing it to 7 mg after a month and then 14 mg. I lost a total of 10 kg over a period of seven–eight months, and now my weight has stabilized. My HbA1C is 5.5.*
>
> *I could feel my appetite shrinking with Rybelsus. My cholesterol levels have improved, though I'm also taking a statin. I eat and drink what I want, and they're not always the healthiest options. The unintended benefit of weight loss has made Rybelsus a good option for me.*

---

*Name changed to protect privacy.

3

Side Effects and How to Manage Them

Many more people die after slipping in the bathroom than in plane crashes. Yet, some people have a fear of flying but not a fear of bathrooms. Any plane crash, with its spectacular visuals, gets much more media attention than a bathroom fall.

It is possible that the next flight you take could crash because planes crash even today. But the benefit of flying outweighs that very low risk. Only one in about 13 million passengers dies in a plane crash.

There is no such thing as zero risk, but flying appears much safer when you look at the data on road accident deaths. Every twenty-six seconds, someone in the world dies of a road accident, yet nobody stays at home.

If some have an irrational fear of flying, others are reckless about flight safety. They don't like to wear seat belts, risking a serious or even fatal head injury in case the flight suddenly experiences air turbulence.

The public conversation on the side effects of GLP-1 drugs is a lot like these two kinds of flight passengers: one who has a fear of flying and the other who thinks that he doesn't need to wear a seat belt.

When any medicine becomes popular among the general public there is often a lot of hype followed by misinformation. The hype leads to self-medication, misuse and avoidable side effects. Negative misinformation leads to exaggeration of a few anecdotes in the media, making many who could benefit from the drug decide against taking it.

We have seen this happen with statins, medicines that reduce cholesterol and prevent clogging of arteries. Every doctor knows how critical statins can be in preventing heart attacks among patients who have heart disease or are at risk of it. The data is solid and irrefutable. Yet the negative, sensationalist, ill-informed media coverage of the side effects of statins makes many patients decide not to take them. A Danish study showed that for every negative nationwide news story about the cholesterol-lowering drug, there was a 9 per cent increased risk of people deciding to stop taking statins.

In a separate study in the UK, it was estimated that at least 2,000 cardiovascular events would occur over the next ten years, which would not have occurred if patients had continued taking statins. Again, this is not to say that everyone should pop statins without medical supervision.

The public tends to divide popular medicines into the binary of good and bad. Any drug that has been approved can be good for us in certain situations. It is the doctor's job to decide if your situation makes the medicine 'good' for you and whether that good outweighs the side effects that you might face. Your doctor will also tell you how to manage those side effects, like the flight crew telling you when it is compulsory to wear seat belts and how to wear an oxygen mask in the rare event that the cabin pressure drops. The one-in-eleven-million possibility of a plane crash should not prevent you from seeing the world.

This is true of many, if not most, medicines. As I said in the introduction, there are people who die of internal bleeding if they take a simple painkiller like aspirin. Does that mean nobody should take aspirin? The benefit of easing pain in millions outweighs the extremely rare risk of internal bleeding. At the same time, this does not mean you should keep popping aspirin all the time. Doing so does increase the risk of side effects. This is why it is important to listen to and follow the doctor's advice on any drug.

I watch with great apprehension how the media, social media and the public is seeing GLP-1 drugs in two extremes. On one hand they are seen as a 'miracle' or a 'magical cure', and on the other extreme, there are endless alarmist articles, videos and WhatsApp forwards describing GLP-1 drugs as being downright dangerous that should be avoided by everyone.

These extremes are reflected in my patients. I see some who just want the prescription and won't listen to anything about what they need to do alongside taking the medicine to avoid side effects and get the best results from their diabetes and obesity management. Then I see patients who clearly need the medicine but are so overcome with the fear of side effects that they are reluctant to take it.

The hype, both positive and negative, is causing harm to the public at large. In the fight against obesity and diabetes, we must be guided by data, science and doctors, not Instagram reels, newspaper articles or overhyped anecdotes.

Prepare for Take-Off

When GLP-1 medicines were first used in human trials in the early 2000s it was seen that people were vomiting all the time. The researchers then tried giving very small doses and found that the side effects became tolerable and subsided with time. Once they went away, patients were given a higher dose to bring about a meaningful decline in their blood sugar levels.

This protocol of starting with a low dose and gradually increasing the dosage is key to managing side effects. The mantra I give my patients is: 'Start low and go slow.'

In Chapter 1, we described the history of GLP-1 drugs and how semaglutide (Ozempic) wasn't the first one. That GLP-1 drugs have been used by patients since 2005 testifies to their general safety. The side effects have also reduced with time. Yet, patients need to be prepared for the gastric and intestinal side effects initially.

Most patients see minimal weight loss and sugar decline in the starting dose of semaglutide (Rybelsus 3 mg, Ozempic 0.25 mg) or tirzepatide (Mounjaro 2.5 mg). This dose is only meant to help the body get used to the drug and get over the side effects. However, for the odd patient, nausea, vomiting, constipation or diarrhoea can be so bad that they need to stop taking the medicine.

Around 15 per cent of my patients taking Rybelsus have had to discontinue taking the pill, most of them due to the side effects. Then there are some lucky ones who don't face any significant side effects from day one! For the vast majority, though, the side effects are significant for a few weeks and then go away. The side effects can sometimes reappear, again temporarily, with each increment in dose.

Data from clinical trials tell us how common the side effects are: 20 per cent faced nausea, 10 per cent had vomiting, 14 per cent had diarrhoea and 5 per cent experienced constipation with Ozempic 1 mg weekly in the SUSTAIN 7 trial.

When used in the full dose of 2.4 mg, nausea was seen in 43.9 per cent (vs 16.1 per cent in the placebo group). Other common side effects were diarrhoea (29.7 per cent vs 15.9 per cent), vomiting (24.5 per cent vs 6.3 per cent) and constipation (24.2 per cent vs 11.1 per cent). The weight loss achieved was not related to the occurrence of gastrointestinal side effects.

Given how easily and frequently they complain of the mildest side effects of diabetes medications, I am sometimes surprised to see patients willing to suffer unpleasant side effects to lose weight. I have some patients who are vomiting every day, running to the bathroom ten times a day, but refuse to give up the medicine. 'It's alright, Doctor, as long as I'm losing weight!'

If the drug does not agree with you, it must be discontinued. In individuals who overdose on the medication or already have weak stomach muscles, like some with long-standing diabetes, the stomach movements can get really slow. This is a condition known as gastroparesis. The stomach is unable to propel the food forward into the intestines, resulting in a stasis of food in the stomach. Such patients have persistent nausea, repeated vomiting, bloating, pain, reflux and even malnutrition as they are unable to eat.

The key is to listen to your body. The risk of something serious happening due to gastrointestinal side effects is higher in those who do not give up the medicine despite intolerable side effects. When your doctor says stop, you must stop.

Everyone's experience of gastrointestinal side effects is different. Some might face constipation, others might experience diarrhoea, and these need to be addressed no differently from when you get constipation and diarrhoea for any other reason.

Drinking plenty of water and eating roughage – high-fibre foods such as vegetables and fruits – will help you minimize constipation. Too much fibre, however, could cause diarrhoea. Probiotics like curd are your friends. High-fat foods, especially fried ones, will worsen your side effects.

Patients who are in a hurry to get the 'magic pill' and are not willing to hear anything to the contrary often make the mistake of not taking dietary measures to manage side effects.

GLP-1 drugs slow down gastric emptying, making you feel full. However, for the same reason, they may also cause constipation, a problem that goes away once your body adjusts to the drug. Constipation is worsened by not eating enough fibre and not drinking enough water. Eating large meals, which the loss of appetite won't let you do anyway, will significantly worsen the gastric side effects. It is best to eat small meals over the course of the day. Aerobic exercises, including walking, may also help relieve constipation.

I often tell my patients that these drugs teach you how to eat. If you stick to small portions of low-fat food, you are much less likely to feel sick. If you violate the norms of eating by indulging in a heavy, fat-rich diet, the GLP-1 will immediately reprimand you by making you feel sick!

Diarrhoea is often caused by fatty and fried foods that your stomach is not ready for yet. While GLP-1 drugs slow down the digestion of food, they may sometimes increase movement in the intestines, aided by changes in gut bacteria.

If your constipation or diarrhoea is out of control, your doctor may give you some medicines or ask you to stop taking GLP-1 drugs. You may take over-the-counter laxatives for constipation, but if you need to take them for more than a few days, it is time to discuss it with your doctor. So far, I have had only two patients who needed to run to the hospital for constipation or diarrhoea.

There is no difference in the nature of side effects whether you take the Rybelsus pill or the Ozempic injection – both are the same drug, semaglutide. However, since the injectable form (Ozempic or Wegovy) delivers a greater amount of medication into the body, which accounts for its greater efficacy, the side effects are also greater. Intuitively, one may feel that a drug given orally will cause more gastrointestinal side effects, but in this case, the side effects are related to the amount of drug reaching our brain via our bloodstream.

Your doctor will prescribe you SOS pills to handle nausea and vomiting. They're both controlled by the brain and are a sign that the drug is effectively reaching the GLP-1 receptors in your brain and likely reducing your desire to eat food. The nausea and vomiting will soon go away, but that loss of appetite will stay, making you lose weight.

Other gastric side effects include burping, which leaves a bad smell and taste in your mouth. This is caused by the slow digestion of food. Water and probiotic-rich foods such as curd will help. Some may experience reflux or heartburn. Avoiding spicy food helps in such cases.

It needs to be reiterated that these gastrointestinal side effects usually go away in a couple of weeks. If they are intolerable, you may need to stop taking GLP-1 drugs. As mentioned above, the side effects can sometimes reappear, again temporarily, with each increment in dose.

Sometimes, patients complain that they're feeling 'weak' on these drugs. This complaint comes mostly from patients with diabetes. Often, it is due to dehydration. Just like one might feel a little weak during fasting, GLP-1 drugs may initially make the patient feel weak due to reduced food intake. The feeling goes away when one gets used to eating less, but having small meals at regular periods might help.

Some patients are able to adjust to the side effects of one GLP-1 drug but not the other. With newer, varied kinds of GLP-1 drugs coming out in the near future, there is still hope for those who are unable to tolerate the gastrointestinal side effects of the currently available GLP-1 drugs.

Dos and Don'ts When You're on GLP-1 Drugs

Here are some dos and don'ts for managing the gastrointestinal side effects, as well as getting the maximum benefit from your GLP-1 medication.

Dos

- Eat slowly and chew well.
- Have smaller portions of food in a meal. Long gaps and huge meals can cause discomfort.
- Walk around for ten to fifteen minutes post-meals instead of immediately lying down.
- In the week after initiation or when starting a higher dose, consume light, soft foods like curd rice, khichdi, well-cooked vegetables and boiled or steamed chicken breast.

- Once drug tolerance improves, the patient can consume regular meals in controlled portions. They can have egg whites, low-fat cheese, Greek yoghurt, fish, nuts, fresh fruits, brown rice, wholegrain bread, quinoa and millets.
- Keep yourself hydrated to prevent constipation.
- Include fresh fruits and vegetables.
- Eat a variety of food from all food groups to keep your diet balanced.
- Eat protein-rich food in each meal. Sources of protein include fish, lean chicken, beans, pulses, tofu, soya, milk and paneer.
- Maintain a regular meal schedule.

Don'ts

- Avoid highly processed fatty foods (chips, namkeen) and deep-fried foods (fried chicken, samosa, mathri). These aggravate gastric side effects like nausea, vomiting and bloating.
- Avoid sugar, honey, jaggery and food products that have these listed in the ingredients list.
- Avoid any food with high-fructose corn syrup in it. Check the labels.
- Avoid liquid calories as these will be absorbed quickly. This includes juices, mocktails, smoothies and high-calorie cream soups.

- Avoid foods that trigger acid reflux like caffeine, refined flour (maida), red chillies and spicy food.
- Avoid very low carbohydrate diets such as the ketogenic diet.
- Limit alcohol and avoid smoking.
- Avoid packaged food like white bread, namkeens, maida, juices (fresh or packaged), rusk, pickles, ketchup, sweets and ice cream.

Change of Taste?

Some patients complain that the joy of food has gone out of their lives. This is again something that usually settles down quickly. Since GLP-1 drugs curb your appetite, some miss the joy of eating in the initial days.

Given the need to make dietary changes to manage the side effects, some are forced to eat healthy foods like salads and fruits they had previously avoided in favour of carbohydrates and processed foods. Studies show that patients taking GLP-1 drugs tend to start choosing healthier foods.

Foods they craved a lot earlier no longer seem tasty to some, but now they want more healthy foods. There is some similarity between the gut and the taste receptors in the tongue, suggesting that GLP-1 signalling may play a role in taste perception. In a recent study, those on semaglutide experienced changes in taste perception and brain activity in response to sweet taste stimuli. It must be mentioned here that some patients on GLP-1 drugs say they now enjoy food more than they used to, since they eat without the cycle of cravings and guilt.

Don't Fear the Injection

While Rybelsus, the daily semaglutide pill, is to be taken orally, Ozempic and Mounjaro are injected into the abdomen. These injectables are similar to the insulin shots taken by diabetes patients. Most people will not see any bleeding, and even if there is any, it will be minor. The injection is subcutaneous (below the skin) and hurts less than a mosquito bite. Adverse skin reactions on the injection site are rare and easily managed.

Hypoglycaemia

Diabetes patients on certain kinds of medication are prone to develop low blood sugar reactions, a condition known as hypoglycaemia. Extreme, untreated hypoglycaemia can be dangerous. Headache, fatigue, dizziness, rapid heartbeat, anxiety and sweating can be some symptoms of hypoglycaemia.

It is crucial to understand that GLP-1 drugs do not produce significant hypoglycaemia by themselves, even when given to those without diabetes. However, their *addition* to the treatment regimen in diabetes can cause hypoglycaemia if the regimen includes oral sulphonylureas or insulin. When I initiate a diabetes patient on GLP-1 drugs, I lower their insulin dose pre-emptively. Still, patients on insulin need to be extra vigilant about their sugar levels because there is no set formula for the amount of insulin dose reduction needed. GLP-1 drugs can sometimes lower sugar levels quite quickly, with or without weight loss.

Loss of Muscle Mass

If you go on a crash diet and rapidly lose a lot of weight, at least 20 per cent of the weight you lose will be muscle mass. It's the same with bariatric surgery and weight loss induced by GLP-1 drugs. Research indicates that these medicines have a positive effect on your muscles and bones, but the weight loss is going to take muscle away with it. What happens when you lose weight but don't maintain muscle mass? Those forty-year-olds who are beginning treatment with GLP-1 drugs today and losing weight without building muscle will find out twenty years later!

Why is muscle mass important? While GLP-1 drugs do not harm the bone directly, weak skeletal muscles weaken bones, apart from giving them poor support. Low muscle mass limits physical activity and makes people more prone to falls and fractures. Fragility fractures, particularly hip fractures, have devastating consequences in the elderly, including a 20 per cent mortality rate within one year of fracture. Low muscle mass also aggravates insulin resistance, thus contributing to obesity and diabetes. Besides, low skeletal muscle mass is associated with greater risk of fatty liver disease.

How can we preserve our muscles while on GLP-1 drugs? To preserve your muscle mass as you lose weight, you must increase your protein intake and do regular strength training. Do not be in a hurry to go up the dosage ladder of GLP-1 drugs. Remember the mantra: Start low and go slow. However, I have had very few patients who take this advice seriously.

As large numbers of people begin to lose weight rapidly with GLP-1 drugs, this issue needs greater attention, especially since Indians tend to have low muscle mass to begin with. This could be due to genetic reasons, but, more importantly, also because of low protein consumption.

We need 0.8 g protein per kg of body weight just to preserve our muscle mass. So, if you weigh 80 kg, you should eat 64 g of protein daily. When you are losing weight, the requirement may go up to 1 g per kg. For most Indians, it is rather challenging to consume this amount of protein.

One whole egg has only 6 g protein, and one katori dal 7 g. Meat eaters find it easier to consume adequate protein. Six pieces of chicken tikka have between 30 and 40 g protein. But even Indians who eat meat don't necessarily have it every day. Whether you are a vegetarian or eat meat, there must be some self-assessment of how much protein you consume from all food sources. Having a protein shake a day, which has around 20–24 g protein, is one way to compensate for the shortfall. Chickpeas (chana), paneer and tofu are some good vegetarian sources of protein.

Consuming adequate protein becomes difficult when GLP-1 drugs curb your appetite and you can't eat much anyway. This is why a planned diet programme is necessary. Some patients make the mistake of thinking they can eat whatever they feel like once the medicine is taking care of their weight and sugar level.

However, increasing protein intake alone is not enough. There has to be resistance and strength training at least twice a week. Walking won't be enough to maintain muscle mass. I recommend that my patients mix resistance training with yoga (two to three days a week each) to experience the benefits of flexibility, mobility, mental health and muscle-building.

Medical advancements – GLP-1 drugs being only one of them – are making people live longer. Yet, poor muscle mass is a top reason for poor quality of life in old age. When you lose weight and regain it, as is often the case with crash diets, the lost muscle mass does not return with the fat tissue. Such yo-yo dieting results in faster degradation of muscle mass over your lifespan. This is why people should avoid misusing GLP-1 drugs for 'quick weight loss before the wedding' and giving them up after the baraatis have gone home. You need muscle mass after the wedding as well.

It would be incorrect to say that loss of muscle mass is a side effect of GLP-1 drugs. It is a side effect of not exercising and not taking adequate protein, both of which affect most Indians, regardless of their body weight and what medicines they are on. This is a major reason why Indians don't win too many medals at the Olympics. Patients taking GLP-1 drugs must see these medicines as part of a wider weight management programme. This includes a diet that is rich in fibre to reduce gastric side effects, adequate protein to preserve muscle mass, regular strength and resistance training to build muscle, along with good sleep and stress management.

'Ozempic Face' and 'Ozempic Butt'

The so-called 'Ozempic face' and 'Ozempic butt' are popular concerns. Ozempic face has been exaggerated in the media and on social media as a problem. It is partly a perception issue: You and the people around you take time to get used to your new face and body as the 'new you'. Any rapid weight loss will have the same effect.

When people with very high BMI lose weight rapidly, they may also develop loose skin. Not everyone will experience this, and the skin often settles with time. Ozempic butt results from fat and muscle loss – again, nothing specifically linked to the drug but a result of weight loss due to any cause.

Once again, the 'start low and go slow' mantra comes into play. The skin needs time to adapt to weight loss, and younger patients will find the adaptation easier. After the weight stabilizes, the skin on the face will also eventually stabilize. Collagen-rich foods like berries, citrus fruits and chicken, along with plenty of water, will help.

Yo-yo changes in weight will make it harder for the skin to adapt each time, so all effort should be made to maintain weight after the rapid weight-loss phase.

Nutritional Deficiencies

Some worry about nutritional deficiencies when they are not eating enough. Common sense dictates that taking multivitamin supplements while on any weight-loss programme, with or without a GLP-1 drug, is a good idea.

Rare Side Effects

Thyroid Cancer

In animal trials of GLP-1 drugs, rodents were found to develop thyroid tumours, some of which were cancerous. In 2023, the European Medicines Agency said it found no link between GLP-1 drugs and an increased risk of any kind of cancer, including thyroid cancer.

Nevertheless, as a precaution, anyone with a family history of medullary thyroid carcinoma, a very rare kind of cancer, should not take GLP-1 drugs. If you have hypothyroidism or hyperthyroidism, this has no bearing on you.

People with a rare, inherited endocrine disorder called MEN type 2 are at risk of tumours in the endocrine system, including thyroid tumours, and are thus on the exclusion list for GLP-1 drugs.

Diabetic Retinopathy

Patients who already have active diabetic retinopathy should not take GLP-1 drugs. Rapid drop in blood sugar levels can sometimes worsen pre-existing diabetic retinopathy, though this effect is likely to be temporary.

We also see this in patients taking insulin. If you do not already have diabetic retinopathy, you don't need to worry about this.

Blurry Vision

In elderly patients, changes in blood sugar levels can also affect the shape of the eye lens, which is less flexible due to age. This causes blurry vision, but it goes away in a few weeks as sugar levels stabilize.

NAION

Two studies, one in the US and one in Denmark, have found that semaglutide increases the incidence of a rare eye condition called NAION, or non-arteritic anterior ischemic optic neuropathy. It occurs when blood flow to the optic nerve is blocked, leading to sudden, painless vision loss in one eye. It could later affect the other eye too. Vision loss can range from moderate to extreme, even causing blindness.

Both studies are observational, meaning that they have found patients taking GLP-1 drugs to be more likely to have NAION. The increase has been seen in patients both with and without diabetes. In one study of hospital records in Denmark, the increased risk was 1.5 to 2.5 patients per 10,000. This was less than what a similar study in the US found.

However, good news has come from a more recent American study. Researchers looked at two groups of people with diabetes: about 120,000 who were prescribed semaglutide and about 220,000 who were prescribed any type of GLP-1 medication. They compared each of these groups to similar people with diabetes who were not taking these medications. There was no significant increase in risk of NAION or ION in patients taking semaglutide or GLP-1 RAs compared to diabetes or high BMI controls. The cumulative incidence of NAION was less than 0.1 per cent up to five years of GLP-1 medication use.

Although the jury is still out on the relationship between GLP-1 drugs and NAION, it is advisable that patients address other factors that increase NAION risk, including managing hypertension, normalizing blood sugar levels, lowering low-density lipoprotein (LDL) or bad cholesterol, quitting smoking, managing sleep apnoea with a continuous positive airway pressure (CPAP) machine, eating an anti-inflammatory diet and exercising.

Before starting GLP-1 drugs, and periodically thereafter as advised by your doctor, an eye check-up is recommended. It is worth noting that diabetes itself is a significant risk factor for eye complications, and improved sugar control with GLP-1 may help enhance long-term eye health.

Allergic Reactions

Allergic reactions to GLP-1 drugs are exceptionally rare, but like with any drug, they can happen. For example, angioedema is an allergy that causes sudden swelling beneath the skin. It commonly affects the face, lips, throat and tongue. If you have such allergies, discuss them with your doctor before starting treatment. If you notice any early symptoms, seek immediate medical help.

Bowel Obstruction

This rare side effect is caused by partial or complete blockage in the intestine, usually in people with underlying gut motility issues. Someone with this condition will have abdominal pain that can be severe, and the patient may not be able to pass stool or gas for days. Such a patient should seek medical attention.

Gastroparesis

This is a weakening of the stomach muscles, also called stomach paralysis, that makes it difficult for your stomach to move food. This can happen if GLP-1 drugs slow down the movement of food excessively. Low doses and slow dosage increases prevent this rare condition. However, this is why people with a history of severe gastrointestinal issues are not to be given GLP-1 drugs.

The symptoms of stomach paralysis may seem similar to the gastric side effects of GLP-1 in the starting period of the drug: nausea, vomiting and bloating. But if these symptoms are severe and don't go away, it could require you to stop taking GLP-1 drugs and seek medical attention.

A significant impact of this can be seen in the reflux of food during anaesthesia administration. Food particles that regurgitate into the throat can enter and get lodged in the lungs. This does not happen normally because of the overnight fast advised before anaesthesia. In patients with underlying gastroparesis, the use of GLP-1 drugs aggravates the condition, and food from several days ago can lie around in the stomach. If you have to undergo surgery, you must inform your surgeon and anaesthetist that you are on GLP-1 drugs. They may advise temporary drug discontinuation before the surgery.

Gallstones

There is a small risk of gall bladder and biliary diseases, particularly the development of gallstones, due to GLP-1 drugs. The risk is greater with higher doses of the drug, especially if you are losing weight too fast.

The odds that you can get gallstones directly as a result of GLP-1 medication are less than one in a hundred. You can reduce this risk further by following the general guidelines on diet and exercise mentioned above.

Kidney Disease

It is advisable to drink enough water and fluids to avoid the rare possibility of dehydration-induced kidney injury if someone has excessive vomiting or diarrhoea with GLP-1 drugs.

Pancreatitis

Sometimes, you may feel some discomfort and bloating in your stomach, especially when you have eaten more than the drug would have liked you to eat. This is the feeling of fullness that comes early because of GLP-1 action in the stomach. However, if there is severe, persistent abdominal pain, do not ignore it. It could be a symptom of pancreatitis. We discussed pancreatitis in the previous chapter – patients with a pre-existing history of pancreatitis should not be given GLP-1 drugs. However, studies also show that GLP-1-induced weight loss actually reduces the risk of pancreatitis in patients. The incidents of pancreatitis are a handful among millions taking this medicine, and even in these cases, it is not yet clearly established whether the drug directly caused it. If you have never had pancreatitis – and if you did, you would know – do not let the word 'pancreatitis' come in the way of taking GLP-1 drugs if your doctor thinks you could benefit from them.

Temporary Hair Loss

Sometimes rapid weight loss can lead to some hair loss, but it is temporary – the hair will return.

Mental Health

Given the known link between obesity and depression, weight loss through GLP-1 drugs should improve mental health, and some trials have indeed proven such improvement. One large scale study analyzed the data of 60 million patients and found no increased suicide risk.

However, there have also been studies to the contrary, including one that has found that GLP-1 drugs may disrupt dopamine activity in individuals who may have pre-existing dopamine disorders, and thus affect mental health adversely.

Side Effects and How to Manage Them

Fear of the Unknown

What are the chances that we might find, say, twenty years from now, that GLP-1 drugs are causing terrible side effects, making us wish we had never used them? This is a highly unlikely scenario, given that GLP-1 drugs have been in clinical use since 2005, exactly twenty years now. Semaglutide itself has been in use for over eight years now.

In a survey carried out in mid-2024 it was found that one in eight adults in the US are taking or have taken a GLP-1 drug. This has resulted in obesity rates now coming down in the US. Millions of people across the world are taking one variant or another. If the side effects outweighed the benefits, we would have known that by now. The side effects of the drug must be compared to the side effects of obesity and diabetes.

A *New York Times* report described how many cardiologists and diabetes specialists in the US are themselves taking these drugs, noticing each other getting thinner at conferences and meetings. That doctors are themselves taking this drug should reassure patients of its safety.

In the next few years, several newer variants of GLP-1 drugs will likely address concerns about side effects. Just as the GLP-1 drugs available today are better than the ones available ten years ago, there will be newer ones which have fewer side effects, provide better sugar control, and variants that may prevent muscle loss.

Given that the risk of side effects is not zero – it never is, for any medicine – the risk does not outweigh the benefit for those who want to take the drug only for cosmetic reasons to lose a couple of kilos. Caution is advised as we proceed with the GLP-1 revolution. This is also why you need to let a doctor decide, based on your medical circumstances and history, whether or not you should be taking a GLP-1 drug.

Takeaway

Many patients starting GLP-1 drugs face gastric or intestinal side effects. They usually subside in a few weeks. If they are intolerable, the patient should discontinue the drug. Serious side effects are very rare, and this risk has to be measured against the vast benefits of treating obesity and diabetes. GLP-1 drugs are safe for most people and a fear of side effects should not hold you back, but make sure you take them under medical supervision.

PATIENT STORY

AMIT JAIN, 50*

I started Ozempic about six months ago with the starting dose of 0.25 mg. It gave me a weight loss of 2.5 kg with no side effects whatsoever, not even mild nausea.

After two months I jabbed myself with a dose of 0.5 mg. Two days later, my side effects were excruciating. Vomiting, loose motions, nausea. They just wouldn't stop. It was so bad I had to be briefly put on a drip.

I went back to 0.25 mg for a while. Later, too afraid to return to 0.5 mg, I turned the injection pen just a little over 0.25 mg, thus taking 0.3 mg. This micro-increase worked. I still had some side effects but the vomiting went away.

For two days after every injection, I face some nausea and loose motions that give way to constipation, but I manage it. Despite the hassle of these side effects, I am still using the drug because I'm desperate to lose weight.

I have lost 4.5 kg in five months despite not being able to increase my dose by much. My weight has decreased from 89.5 kg to 85 kg, and my target is 68 kg. My wife is also on Ozempic. She has reached the 1.5 mg dose, has no

---

*Name changed to protect privacy.

side effects, and has lost 7 kg. My daughter has also lost a lot of weight on Rybelsus.

Apart from the weight loss, one good thing has been that it has reduced our desire to drink alcohol. I no longer drink daily but only socially. My wife is unable to have a single drink. However, it has, strangely, given me a sugar craving I never had.

I started putting on weight when I was around thirty-five. It started with a beer belly. Diets have on and off helped me reduce weight, but it comes back. I'm hoping the side effects will subside and I can make the drug work better for me.

4

The GLP-1 Journey

A few weeks into GLP-1 medication, when the side effects go away and patients lose a few kilos of weight, they tell me how good they feel, more alert and agile. Some of them tried to lose weight for years without any success. Now, finally, something worked. They're ecstatic. They have finally crossed the Rubicon into the weight-loss zone.

Feeling good about yourself is important. With GLP-1 medication, those with diabetes begin to see how they need fewer medications and how their blood sugar levels are coming down to less alarming levels.

Yet, the excitement of weight loss can lead to many mistakes in the GLP-1 journey. You must talk to your doctor about what to expect in the next few weeks.

The first mistake is to start these medicines with unrealistically high expectations. Patients who think they're going to lose 20 kg in three months will not only

be disappointed, but will also make mistakes they may later regret.

One must be ready for potential disappointment. Some patients may respond minimally or not at all. I have patients who have lost only 6–7 kg on high doses of Mounjaro, and some who have lost 20 kg on the same doses. The odd ones may not lose anything at all (less than 3 kg).

More studies are needed to explain why some people are 'non-responders', losing less than 5 per cent of their baseline weight. In clinical trials, 10–15 per cent people have been found to be non-responders. The reasons could include genetic and hormonal variations, differences in brain activity, untreated sleep apnoea, stress, anti-depressants, steroids and contraceptives.

People with diabetes tend to lose less weight with GLP-1 drugs than those without diabetes. It has been suggested that diabetes background medications may promote weight gain. Other factors that could account for less weight loss in people with diabetes could be greater food intake due to fear of low blood sugar, altered gut microbiota and a genetic background that predisposes them to gain weight. They may have had long-standing obesity or may be less likely to exercise.

The proportion of people who do not see results on GLP-1 drugs has been coming down with each new variant over the years, and in the future, there will be many more options.

Starting Dose

GLP-1 medications are currently expensive and not easily available. This will change within the next two years. As mentioned in Chapter 1, Rybelsus, the first and only GLP-1 receptor agonist in pill form, was approved in India in January 2022. It is currently approved for diabetes but not for weight loss. However, doctors may prescribe it off-label for weight loss if the patient has other obesity-related health conditions such as sleep apnoea, hypertension, joint inflammation, and so on. The average weight loss reported with Rybelsus is in the range of 3 to 4 kg. In our recently published data, the mean weight loss achieved by Indian patients with diabetes over six months was about 4 per cent of baseline weight. Remember, Rybelsus is essentially an anti-diabetes drug that provides the additional benefit of weight loss.

Mounjaro was launched in India in March 2025 and Wegovy is expected soon. Some of my patients have been procuring them from abroad.

Rybelsus 3 mg daily pill is the starting dose. The pill has to be taken with some precautions to be effective. Most of this 3 mg gets metabolized and very little reaches your bloodstream. Hence, patients must take it with half a glass of water first thing in the morning and then eat or drink nothing – not even water – for forty-five minutes.

You are not expected to lose any weight on a dose as low as this. It is only meant to make you get used to the drug and get past the gastric side effects seen in many patients. Nausea is the most common side effect. In the previous chapter, we discussed side effects and how to manage them in great detail. You must be prepared for the side effects.

Unlike its effect on weight loss, the effect on sugar control is apparent earlier, and stays even after the weight loss stabilizes. However, some patients may also lose weight in the first month, sometimes as much as 2–3 kg.

This is when patients start making mistakes. Some may have a friend who lost a lot of weight on the starting dose; why are *they* not losing any weight? Sometimes patients put up with overpowering side effects just because they are losing weight. Sometimes they lose 1–2 kg and then the weight loss stops, so in a hurry to lose weight, they jump to the next dose – 7 mg – without consulting the doctor.

Some physicians advise stepping up the dose to 7 mg after 10–15 days if the patient does not report side effects. **The recommended protocol for the new GLP-1 drugs, semaglutide (Rybelsus, Ozempic, Wegovy) and tirzepatide (Mounjaro, Zepbound), is that the patient should stay on each dose for at least four weeks. Increasing doses faster than that is usually a bad idea for several reasons.**

For one, early escalation increases the chances of stomach- and intestine-related side effects. Most individuals require some time to adjust to the medication. The concept of a slow increase in dose is based on minimizing the abdominal side effects.

Second, there could be other side effects too. People with diabetes, in particular, need to be careful about hypoglycaemia and should adjust other medicines according to changes in blood sugar levels. There are several side effects caused by rapid weight loss, whether through GLP-1 medications or lifestyle measures. The rare eye-related complications reported with GLP-1 drugs are also likely related to rapid control of blood glucose.

Third, patients choosing early escalation do not maximize the potential gains from each dose. What looked like a 'plateau' may not have been a plateau. Maybe you could have lost more weight on that dose if you had persisted with it for another week or two.

Fourth, as stated in the previous chapter, the faster the weight loss, the more muscle you lose. Instead of focusing on increasing protein intake despite appetite suppression and doing strength training, some patients get glued to the weighing scale to see if they lost some more on a daily basis.

Fifth, there is a small risk of nutrient deficiencies due to rapid weight loss since you're eating less. This, however, is usually managed well with a multivitamin or other supplements, depending on blood reports.

Sixth, some patients, particularly those with diabetes, complain of feeling weak or fatigued. This also happens sometimes because of rapid weight loss and sugar control. Often, diet changes and hydration help, but not increasing dosage very quickly is wise for this reason as well.

Most patients want to lose weight quickly. Very few come to me saying they'd like to lose it gradually. Remember the mantra: **START LOW AND GO SLOW!**

Dose Escalation

As stated earlier, for Rybelsus, the initial dose is 3 mg, which typically does not produce much weight loss. The next dose is 7 mg, in which some weight loss is expected, and lastly 14 mg. Patients may realize that they don't have a higher dose to escalate to after 14 mg, while their goal weight is still some distance away. Recent research has shown that 25 and 50 mg doses may be more effective and equally safe. I won't be surprised if they are available in a couple of years.

Like Rybelsus, Ozempic and Wegovy are also semaglutide, but in the form of a weekly self-injection. They free you from the need to take a pill first thing every morning and then wait for forty-five minutes for even a sip of water. With their ability to achieve higher blood levels of semaglutide, injectable preparations are superior to Rybelsus when it comes to weight loss. The highest currently used dose of Rybelsus is roughly equivalent to a 1 mg weekly dose of Ozempic. With Ozempic, patients can go up to 2 mg weekly, and with Wegovy up to 2.4 mg. Remember again that all three contain exactly the same drug, made by the same company. **Patients taking Ozempic or Wegovy can lose an average of 10–15 per cent of their total body weight as compared to about 4–5 per cent with Rybelsus. Do not make the mistake of overdosing: We must follow the current guidelines on what is safe.**

Mounjaro and Zepbound both contain tirzepatide, which acts via two pathways, GLP-1 and GIP, as explained in Chapter 1. Like Ozempic, tirzepatide is administered by a weekly self-injection, and has proven to be a highly effective drug, surpassing the average weight loss achieved with Ozempic or Wegovy. Losing 20 per cent of baseline weight has been reported with Mounjaro.

Like the oral Rybelsus, GLP-1 injectables medications are typically uptitrated every four weeks. The injections come in preloaded syringes or vials and are easily self-injected.

What should be a patient's reasonable target weight, and when is a good time to increase the dosage? The answer will vary from person to person, depending on their medical needs. Thus, this decision is best made in consultation with your doctor and not by yourself. There have been reports of patients landing up in hospital because they were self-medicating, initiating therapy on a higher dose than recommended and, at times, taking whatever dosage they could find.

There are patients who reach a reasonable BMI but want to increase their dosage only for cosmetic reasons. I discourage this. Sometimes I face the opposite problem. There are patients who need to lose more weight for better health outcomes, but they think they've lost enough and don't wish to increase the dosage.

The speed of weight loss should be a truly clinical judgement, depending on the individual medical circumstances of each patient. An old rule of thumb in the pre-GLP-1 era was to aim for a weight loss of 2–4 kg a month. If the drug continues to work for six months, it can result in 12–24 kg of weight loss!

In general, the guiding principle is to reach the highest tolerated dose. The idea is not just to maximize weight loss but also to gain other health benefits of GLP-1 drugs, as explained in Chapter 7. There are, however, several caveats. If a patient has lost more than expected weight on a particular dose, I ask them to continue on that dose for some more time and not be in a hurry. If a patient is nearing target weight and still continuing to lose weight, I'll suggest they give their dosage some more time before considering an escalation. But if they are a long way off from goal weight or respond poorly to lower doses, the considerations might change. Obviously, looking at other health indicators, such as gastrointestinal side effects, sugar control, laboratory reports, and muscle mass, is important as well.

How effective the drug will be for an individual can be a bit of a lottery!

There has been a worldwide shortage of the newer GLP-1 drugs, which is now getting better. As you can see from the table below, there are currently three doses of Rybelsus, four of Ozempic and five of Mounjaro. While Wegovy is the same molecule as Ozempic, it is available in slightly higher doses.

Table 2: Available doses of GLP-1 drugs

Sl No	Rybelsus (oral semaglutide)	Ozempic (semaglutide)	Wegovy (semaglutide)	Mounjaro (tirzepatide)
1	3 mg	0.25 mg	0.25 mg	2.5 mg
2	7 mg	0.5 mg	0.5 mg	5 mg
3	14 mg	1 mg	1 mg	7.5 mg
4	–	2 mg	1.7 mg	10 mg
5	–	–	2.4 mg	15 mg

There is a new trend among the American youth to 'microdose' with GLP-1 drugs. They don't turn the pen fully and inject very small quantities. While the impact of 'microdosing' has not been studied, it should not cause any harm, and may even minimize side effects. However, even if microdosing helps lose some weight, it is unclear that the benefits of these drugs for overall health outcomes will be the same.

Dealing with Missed Doses

What do you do if you miss taking a dose on the seventh day? If the next dose is more than two days away, you may take the dose immediately. Let's say you take the dose every Monday, but you were travelling and couldn't get hold of the drug. You return home on Thursday. Now, the next dose is scheduled for Monday. Never mind, take your missed dose on Thursday and the next one on Monday as scheduled.

However, if the next dose is less than 48 hours away – let's say you returned home only on Saturday night, then wait until Monday to take your dose as per your weekly schedule.

If you missed two or more doses in a row, then restart on your scheduled day of the week. In such cases, restarting may sometimes cause excessive gastrointestinal side effects. To avoid them, you may start with a lower dose than the one you were last taking.

Maximize Your Loss

The other factors determining how much weight you can lose on each dose are diet and exercise. Yes, **the drugs curb your appetite and make you eat less, but what you eat is also important. Focusing on fibre and protein while going easy on high-fat, deep-fried foods, sugar and carbohydrates will help accelerate weight loss.** To improve tolerability you can escalate doses according to the recommended protocol, eat small meals, drink plenty of water and stay away from the keto diet or other high-fat diets when on GLP-1.

There is no food that is totally disallowed because one is on GLP-1 medication. Some patients become especially careless about what they eat because the overall calorie deficit makes them lose weight anyway, so they don't bother about trying to eat healthy. This approach can affect how much weight they lose on the drug as well as impact other health outcomes. Working with a nutritionist will help them understand their individual dietary needs better.

Fibre plays a key role in supporting gut health, as well as helping the body absorb essential minerals and vitamins. It helps reduce glucose spikes, as it absorbs and binds it. You need vegetables, not just for fibre, but also for antioxidants. Too much fibre, however, creates its own problems when one is on GLP-1 drugs, such as bloating and diarrhoea.

Protein also helps with satiety, making you feel full on fewer calories, and helps preserve and build muscle mass. It thus reduces the amount of refined carbohydrates being consumed. Protein also prevents glucose spikes. I have rarely seen any Indian patient consume too much protein. However, attempting a very high protein diet with little fibre can lead to constipation.

If I were to recommend an ideal meal for patients on GLP-1 medication, it would be a chicken or paneer salad with a variety of vegetables, maybe some berries and nuts, and a low-sugar salad sauce. If there was one food I would advise patients on GLP-1 to avoid, it is fried food. Fried foods are heavy and filling in a situation where your stomach is already slowing down digestion, making it difficult for you to eat much else.

Another way to maximize your loss is to exercise, including cardio and strength training. The latter will help increase your basal metabolic rate, or BMR, the calories your body burns to maintain basic functions like breathing and blood circulation. The calories burnt through cardio exercises like walking are over and above the BMR. While losing weight, your BMR comes down because your body now needs to burn fewer calories for those basic functions. This comes in the way of additional weight loss.

Strength training helps overcome this effect, and provides benefits of healthy muscle mass such as joint support and reduced insulin resistance. While lifting weights against gravity, muscles contract against resistance and become bigger and stronger. Muscle tissue burns more calories than fat, and muscle gain with strength training increases your BMR.

Aerobic exercises will help more than muscle-building with short-term weight loss; muscle-building will be crucial in long-term weight management. Aerobic exercises are important to make your heart healthier, pump more blood and keep the arteries unclogged. Regular exercise, both cardio and strength, helps suppress appetite.

Breaking the Plateau

Diet and exercise can particularly help when you feel a slight return of appetite, as the brain builds tolerance to the dose, and therefore, weight loss slows down.

Every time you start a new dose, there is a window of a few weeks until you build tolerance for it and stop losing weight, and those mild gastric side effects disappear. Maximizing your weight loss in this window through some extra diet and exercise effort can be helpful. This is also when you are losing muscle along with body fat; hence, strength training is a must.

In other words, whether it is for side effects, maximizing weight loss, or overcoming a weight-loss plateau, seeing these drugs as only a part of your weight management programme is a must. The other parts are diet, exercise, good sleep and stress management. It is a package that should start together from the first day of the drug.

Stress, poor sleep, not drinking enough water, lack of exercise, and eating the wrong foods, especially sugar, will reduce both the amount and the speed of weight loss. Patients who see GLP-1 medication as a 'magical cure', as if they don't need to work on their lifestyle any more, will underutilize the potential of the drug. Too many mangoes could slow down your weight loss even if the medication allows you the appetite to eat them!

Maintenance Dose

Many patients come to me thinking these drugs are a quick fix and are surprised to hear that it will take about a year even to reach their goal weight and they may have to continue the drug for much longer, possibly lifelong.

Obesity is a chronic disease that needs lifelong management in the same way as diabetes, hypertension and heart disease. Reaching the target weight on GLP-1 drugs is not the end of the journey. It may well be the beginning. Despite reaching the target weight, patients have to continue the drug. That is what the research says: Stopping the drug brings back that old appetite, that 'food noise', and the weight returns. One school of thought says that patients will have to be on these drugs lifelong, but there's another emerging school of thought that says patients should commit to the drug for at least two years and then try to taper it off.

It is difficult for patients to go off the GLP-1 medication completely unless they create an altogether new lifestyle with a low-calorie diet, regular exercise, better sleep and stress management. Gradual de-escalation of doses allows us to take a call about this while avoiding sudden weight swings.

Once the target weight has been reached, I ask my patients to reduce the dosage by one level. If they add a kilo or so after that, it's alright. If they suddenly add 3 to 4 kg, I suggest they return to the earlier, higher dose.

My biggest fear is that some patients might use the drugs on and off, losing and gaining weight all the time rather than staying at a stable weight point. This yo-yo in weight makes it progressively more challenging to lose weight in subsequent attempts. Besides, when you regain weight, it will mainly be fat – muscle mass will remain low.

I say two things to patients who worry about the long-term effects of GLP-1 drugs. First, you will soon be taking better versions of these drugs, which may be more tailored to your specific medical situation, have fewer side effects and greater efficacy. We discuss these future drugs in Chapter 9.

Second, even if you stop it – under supervision – and gradually regain some weight, you would still have gained good health for a few years. Obesity and diabetes cause a plethora of diseases and heart conditions that impair quality of life. Even five years of good health added to a patient's life will reduce or delay the risk of heart attacks, liver disease and other complications.

Hard evidence is still lacking about whether to continue a lifelong high dose, move to a maintenance dose, or stop the drug altogether. Physicians use their clinical judgement to decide the course of action.

Scientists have been trying for a long time to treat obesity with medication, but the path of anti-obesity drugs is littered with failures. Until semaglutide came around, any drugs that caused weight loss didn't seem to work beyond six months. GLP-1 drugs continue to produce weight loss for at least a year and maintain it afterwards. Finally, we have something that gives lasting results. People who have struggled with obesity for years and decades know how difficult it is to prevent body fat from returning once you lose it with a lot of effort. The GLP-1 medication journey is different: Staying on the drug makes sure the weight doesn't return.

Takeaway

Start GLP-1 drugs with a low dose to manage the side effects. The dosage is increased gradually as the weight loss and sugar control plateau and side effects subside. The desire to lose weight very fast can be counter-productive. Patients must avoid dosage mistakes and increase their dosage in consultation with their doctor. The golden mantra is START LOW AND GO SLOW.

PATIENT STORY

SANJAY AGGARWAL, 59

I have had diabetes for thirty years now and have been visiting Dr Mithal for the last twenty years. Around 2022, I started taking a GLP-1 drug, dulaglutide, under the brand name Trulicity. Along with lifestyle changes in diet and exercise, it helped me lose around 10 per cent of my weight in the course of a year and a half. More importantly, it helped a lot to bring down my HbA1c. It used to be around 7.5–8 per cent before Trulicity, and the drug helped bring it down to around 7. But I continued to be on multiple diabetes medicines, including insulin. My insulin requirement came down marginally with Trulicity. I tolerated the side effects well, hardly facing any nausea.

Around six months ago I switched from Trulicity to Mounjaro. I had high expectations from an expensive medicine that I sourced from Dubai since it was until recently not available in India. Unfortunately, I have lost only 3 kg on Mounjaro in six months despite reaching the highest available dose, 15 mg. I was 118 kg before I began Trulicity, and 105 kg when I began Mounjaro. Now I'm 102 kg.

However, the diabetes control has been phenomenal. My HbA1c now hovers around 5.6. Overall, my parameters look a lot better, and Dr Mithal told me it also has a protective effect on my organs. Some of my other diabetes medications have reduced as well. With Dr Mithal's supervision, I am slowly tapering off other medicines, including insulin.

I'm still hopeful of losing more weight. I feel my energy levels have come down a bit since I started taking Mounjaro. I have been a disciplined eater, and have been working with nutritionists. Mounjaro has majorly suppressed my appetite. I eat breakfast and then don't feel like eating until dinner.

Mounjaro has given fabulous results for so many people but I don't know why it hasn't resulted in the expected weight loss for me. I am looking forward to newer GLP-1 drugs in the future.

5

The ABCD of Weight Gain

The World Health Organization (WHO) classified obesity as a disease as long ago as 1997. However, even today, not many think of it as a disease – honestly, not even many doctors. Excess fat is seen as only a condition that leads to many diseases but not as a disease by itself.

This view is beginning to change with the success of GLP-1 drugs in addressing obesity. Now that we have a medicine for it, people are more likely to see it as a disease.

In 2017, the American Association of Clinical Endocrinologists and the American College of Endocrinology coined a new term to describe obesity: adiposity-based chronic disease or ABCD. The idea is to define obesity accurately and to phase out the term 'obesity' in clinical practice because of the societal stigma associated with it. Equally important is the 'D' in the new term – disease.

The ABCD of Weight Gain

The term 'ABCD' also helps emphasize the limitations of BMI in understanding the extent to which a person is affected by body fat. As mentioned in a previous chapter, BMI only tells us about weight in relation to height – it doesn't tell us how much of that weight is fat, how much of it is around critical internal organs (visceral fat), and the extent to which it causes hormonal or immunological damage to the patient.

Adipose tissue stores energy to use it later when more energy is needed. It provides thermal insulation to maintain body temperature, pads and protects internal organs from injury, helps regulate key metabolic hormones, and has immune cells that respond to injury and infections.

However, putting on weight and accumulating more adipose tissue than you need is like having too much of a good thing. We need to understand how excessive adipose tissue harms our bodies, even in the early stages of the disease, when people think, 'I'm only a little overweight, it's alright, everyone is these days.' Even at this early stage, the damage begins. It has been difficult to make people understand the insidious impact of even being slightly overweight. I'm often in a situation where I have to explain to someone with a BMI of 27 why he or she needs to lose weight even though their blood sugar, blood pressure and cholesterol are under control with medication.

Others desperately want to get thin for cosmetic reasons, despite being normal weight. I see both kinds in my clinic.

Forest Fire

Adipose tissue isn't just passively sitting there. It is doing things. One of the things it does is release pro-inflammatory cytokines.

Inflammation is a bodily response to injury and infection. If you get a cut, it won't heal without inflammation. But chronic inflammation is like an endless low-grade fire ravaging a forest. It begins to slowly and steadily damage your organs.

This is particularly the case with visceral fat inside your belly and around the internal organs. It is metabolically more active and secretes more inflammatory cytokines, leading to chronic inflammation.

'Viscera' refers to the body's internal organs in the chest, abdomen and pelvic cavities. These include heart, lungs, oesophagus, windpipe, stomach, intestines, liver, gall bladder, pancreas, kidneys, bladder, uterus, ovaries and prostate gland, among others. **The body begins to deposit fat close to these organs partly because, in times of stress and starvation, it can access the stored energy easily. That is why belly fat is the easiest to put on.**

The ABCD of Weight Gain

The damage to these organs from inflammatory cytokines does not occur overnight. It is a gradual process. Once it begins, you need to put the fire out or at least not let it become bigger. Many are unable to douse it, and it grows bigger over decades.

The more weight you put on, the more adipose tissue is concentrated around your belly and the greater the inflammation. You will start seeing a rise in inflammatory markers in your blood reports. By reducing inflammation, it reduces your relative risk of numerous diseases that are, in turn, caused by ABCD.

The body collects fat for a rainy day when there may be food scarcity. It likes to accumulate it close to the critical body organs found in the abdomen. This explains why people, especially men, start putting on weight in their bellies first. The good news is that visceral fat is also usually the first to go when you lose weight. Since this fat is around your organs and not visible outwardly, the initial few kilos of weight loss is not apparent before the mirror. This is also why moderate weight loss goes a long way. If you lose only 5 kg and not 15 kg, it is still highly beneficial for your health outcomes.

Up to a certain age, women are relatively more protected from the impact of obesity due to the hormone oestrogen. This is why they tend to put on more weight on their thighs and hips initially, whereas, in men, it is often in the abdomen, where it is most harmful for internal organs. This is also partly why women live longer than men. However, this protective effect goes away in high BMIs as well as after menopause, when women see a redistribution of body fat, increased visceral fat and loss of muscle mass.

When the Key Can't Open the Lock

Among the early effects of chronic inflammation is insulin resistance. Your body produces insulin, but it is not working as it should.

Our cells need glucose for energy. They are locked, and insulin's job is to open the lock and let glucose enter. However, excessive fat tissue and cytokines block the way for insulin, strengthening the lock. It can no longer open that lock. This is called insulin resistance.

The pancreas jumps into action, producing more insulin. As you keep gaining weight, the pancreas can't produce enough insulin to make all the glucose enter the cells effectively. That's when the levels of glucose in your blood start rising.

When insulin resistance starts initially, your blood sugar levels may still be normal. But over time, the pancreas just can't keep up, and eventually, sugar levels rise, resulting in diabetes.

Remember, insulin's job is to get glucose into blood cells, thus helping you convert glucose into fat. So, the increased insulin levels reduce your blood sugar but increase your adipose tissue.

Insulin spikes cause sugar crashes, making you hungrier. The hormone leptin does try to fight this situation by signalling fullness to the brain, making you eat less. However, diets high in sugar, starch and saturated fat can result in resistance to leptin.

This vicious cycle of insulin and glucose affects the body from head to toe, and you accumulate more fat tissue. We can fight this vicious cycle with lifestyle changes and now medication.

Head to Toe

When people start putting on weight, there comes a time when their metabolism can't keep up. They start experiencing fatigue, greater cravings for carbohydrates and sugar, energy crashes, and even difficulty focusing (brain fog). Increasingly, they find it difficult to lose weight.

Brain

Obesity has been linked to increased cognitive decline, memory loss and a reduction in grey-matter volume. It has been found that people in their early forties with the highest levels of abdominal fat were nearly three times more likely to develop dementia and Alzheimer's disease – in which brain cells begin to die and the brain shrinks – by their mid-seventies to early eighties. The link between excess fat and Alzheimer's disease is so clear that it has been called 'obesity of the brain'. GLP-1 drugs are showing great potential in alleviating Alzheimer's in ongoing trials.

With time, obesity also increases the risk of brain stroke. Being overweight increases the risk of stroke by 22 per cent, and if you are obese, that risk increases by 64 per cent. Central obesity correlates better with stroke risk, and the correlation is stronger in the middle-aged population rather than the elderly. The reason for increased stroke risk in obesity is related to high blood pressure, heart disease, high cholesterol and type 2 diabetes.

Sleep

Fat tissue starts depositing around the neck, physically narrowing the upper airway. This obstructs normal breathing during sleep (which is why people snore), causing a condition known as sleep apnoea. Fat tissue can even accumulate on the tongue, making it larger and heavier, and thus more prone to collapsing back into the airway during sleep.

The brain prevents such patients from going into deep sleep because they need some alertness to not altogether stop breathing. When sleep apnoea becomes severe, patients may start waking up in the middle of the night and feeling excessively thirsty. It's the brain waking them up to enable them to breathe. Even apart from apnoea, obesity is linked to poorer quality of sleep.

Skin and Hair

Insulin resistance causes dark skin patches with a velvety texture, typically in body folds like the neck, armpits and groin. This is called acanthosis nigricans. With weight loss and sugar control, these patches lighten but may never fully go away.

Obesity also makes other skin problems, such as skin tags, acne, and fungal and bacterial infections in skin folds, more likely.

Additionally, studies have shown a correlation between high BMI, hair thinning and hair loss, particularly male-pattern balding.

Lungs

The impact of obesity on lung function is related to the mechanical and inflammatory aspects of obesity.

Fat deposits in the chest make it harder to expand and contract the lungs to breathe, thus affecting lung function and often lowering blood oxygen levels. In someone with a very high BMI, it is not uncommon to see fatigue and breathlessness. American women with high levels of visceral fat were found in a study to be 37 per cent more likely to develop asthma than women with smaller waists – even if their weight was normal.

This could be because of inflammatory effects in the airway. The pressure of fat tissue on the lungs also worsens breathlessness. Inflammation begins to damage lung tissue, leading to a condition called fibrosis.

Heart

This muscular organ sustains life by pumping blood to deliver oxygen to the body through a network of blood vessels. Inflammation, high blood sugar and high blood pressure begin to damage the smooth inner layer of blood vessels, called the endothelial lining. The rising LDL cholesterol gets deposited on its arterial walls due to endothelial damage. These deposits thicken to form plaques, narrowing and ultimately choking the artery. The clogged arteries don't let your heart receive blood supply; without blood, the heart muscle is deprived of oxygen and nutrients, resulting in heart attacks. A large study of European women aged forty-five to seventy-nine concluded that those with the biggest waists had more than double the risk of developing heart disease. In healthy, non-smoking women, every two inches of additional waist size raised the risk for cardiovascular disease by 10 per cent.

Obesity damages the heart in numerous other ways too. The heart has to pump more blood to support all that additional body weight. Over time, this strain on the heart also weakens it.

Blood Pressure

Obesity is a leading cause of chronically elevated blood pressure. Extra body fat requires more oxygen and nutrients, necessitating the heart to pump more blood. This hard work increases the pressure exerted inside the blood vessels. Uncontrolled blood pressure raises the risk of heart attacks, brain stroke, kidney failure and vision loss.

Liver

The body's largest internal organ helps digest food, extract nutrients, cleanse the blood of toxins, and a lot more. When more than 5–10 per cent of the weight of the liver is adipose tissue, inflammation starts to damage liver cells. This comes in the way of the liver doing its job.

There was a time when liver disease was perceived to be primarily an alcohol-related problem. But with rising obesity, we see wide prevalence of what is popularly known as fatty liver disease and is now in medical terminology known as MASLD or metabolic dysfunction-associated steatotic liver disease. Often it has no symptoms, though it may cause fatigue, weakness and abdominal discomfort.

Obesity increases the risk of elevated liver enzymes by two to three times, and the risk of fatty liver by three to fifteen times, depending on the degree of obesity.

Unchecked, MASLD may lead to extensive scarring and fibrosis of the liver, resulting in cirrhosis and even liver cancer. Clinically, it can present as jaundice, severe itching, fluid retention and altered consciousness, and may be fatal. Not all with MASLD go down this path; genetic factors may determine the propensity to develop chronic liver disease.

Bones and Joints

Extra body fat increases the load on our joints, especially knees, hips and lower back. This accelerates cartilage wear and tear, increasing the risk of osteoarthritis. Inflammation from fat tissue also directly contributes to cartilage breakdown.

Abdominal fat leads to poor posture, a condition known as lordosis, which can cause chronic lower back pain. Obesity makes bones weaker directly through inflammation. Poor vitamin D levels, often seen in obese individuals, make it worse. This increases the risk of falls and fractures.

Obesity also raises the levels of uric acid, causing gout, manifesting itself in pain in toes, ankles and knees.

Obese individuals also tend to have pain in the feet while walking, caused by flattening of their feet arches and plantar fasciitis. They're also more likely to sprain their ankles.

Gastrointestinal Health

Overweight and obese people often complain of excessive burping, heartburn or flatulence. These are symptoms of GERD and acid reflux. This happens because visceral fat increases abdominal pressure, pushing stomach acid into the oesophagus, the tube that carries food from the mouth to the stomach.

Obesity also alters the gut microbiome, promoting harmful microbes that increase insulin resistance and inflammation. Other conditions, such as chronic constipation, leaky gut and gallstones, are also linked to obesity.

Immunity

Due to inflammation and hormone dysregulation, obesity reduces overall immunity to bacterial and viral infections, and increases the severity of their impact once you get them. Studies have shown that obese individuals were at significantly higher risk of hospitalization and death due to Covid-19.

Cancer

Obesity is linked to a significantly increased risk of some kinds of cancer. These include breast cancer in postmenopausal women, colon cancer (especially in men), endometrial, oesophageal, kidney, gall bladder, ovarian and prostate cancers. The increased cancer risk is again largely because of inflammation and hormonal alterations.

Sexual Health

Obesity disrupts sex hormones in both men and women.

In men, it lowers testosterone levels, leading to decreased libido, erectile dysfunction and reduced sperm quality, making it harder for their partners to conceive. Inflammation and insulin resistance reduce blood flow to the genitalia.

In women, obesity disrupts sexual and reproductive health by interfering with hormone balance and menstrual cycles. Excess body fat increases oestrogen levels and insulin resistance, which can lead to irregular periods, PCOS and difficulty in conceiving. Polycystic ovary syndrome is a hormonal disorder that affects women, causing irregular periods, excessive hair growth, and acne. It occurs when the ovaries produce too many androgens (male hormones), which disrupts ovulation and can lead to small fluid-filled sacs (cysts) in the ovaries. It raises the risk of diabetes, infertility and other long-term health issues if left unmanaged.

Obesity also raises the risk of pregnancy-related complications, such as gestational diabetes and high blood pressure, affecting both the mother and baby. Additionally, it can lower libido and impact sexual satisfaction due to hormonal changes and reduced blood flow.

Skeletal Muscle

The muscles around our skeleton enable movement and maintain posture. Obesity weakens muscles by increasing strain, reducing strength and promoting muscle loss over time. The extra weight forces muscles, especially in the legs and the back, to work harder, causing fatigue and increasing the risk of injury.

Chronic inflammation and insulin resistance in obesity also interfere with muscle repair and growth, making them weaker.

Mental health

Like much else with obesity, mental health and fat accumulation is a vicious cycle. People with high body fat are much more likely to be depressed and/or have chronic anxiety. This is not just because of body-image issues and the social stigma associated with obesity. It is also because obesity has been linked to poor mood regulation and changes in the brain caused by inflammation. Depression and anxiety often make people overeat, creating a vicious cycle. Mental health conditions can also come in the way of getting enough physical activity that might help with weight management.

Prevention Is Better than Cure

A disease is a disorder or abnormal condition that affects the structure or function of an organism. By that definition, obesity is a disease. It may not be an exaggeration to call it a meta-disease as it is the main driver of non-communicable diseases today. The WHO says, 'Overweight is a condition of excessive fat deposits. Obesity is a chronic complex disease defined by excessive fat deposits that can impair health.'

A shift in public perception to recognize obesity as a disease would have far-reaching consequences. For one, people may not take it lightly when they first start putting on weight. This is when the chances of fighting obesity with lifestyle modifications are the highest.

There would be nothing better than people not needing GLP-1 medications at all. After all, prevention is better than cure.

Takeaway

Obesity is a meta-disease, the mother of most non-communicable diseases. It causes other diseases from head to toe. It is important to start seeing obesity as a disease and not merely a condition that causes diseases. The main mechanism through which obesity starts harming the body is chronic inflammation. The most harmful fat is around the critical organs in the abdomen.

PATIENT STORY

VARUN TULI, 42

I was underweight as an infant, and so I was overfed. I became overweight when I was around ten years old. My asthma medications contributed to it as well. Since then, there have been three periods in my life when I have lost considerable weight.

The first was when I was in college. I went on the Atkins diet, in which you try not to eat any carbs. I also did a lot of exercise. Losing weight helped me get more attention from women, which was the purpose. But it did not last long and the weight returned.

A few years later I went on the South Beach diet, in which you eat only healthy carbs – no potatoes, sugar or alcohol. This worked, and the results lasted a few years. But then I got married and got into the restaurant business. My work needed me to travel and try restaurants across the world. We also set up a catering business that operates across the world.

My weight went up to 127.5 kg. Surprisingly, I didn't have many issues, my HbA1c was around 5.7, and my blood test reports were alright. The only major problem was fatty liver. When it almost reached grade 3, the gastroenterologist referred me to Dr Mithal, who was in no hurry to put me on a GLP-1 drug.

He first put me on Jardiance (an SGLT2 inhibitor) and made me work with a nutritionist for a structured diet plan. I lost 10 kg with this approach. Thereafter, he felt the time was right to begin with the GLP-1 approach.

I have lost 23 kg on Mounjaro in a year. I would like to lose another 17. I have been taking the highest dose, 15 mg, for two months now and am still losing weight, albeit slowly. Coupled with lifestyle modifications, I think I can get there. I'm glad I have lost weight slowly yet steadily.

Blood test reports show my liver is now in excellent shape. My HbA1c has come down to 5.1, which surprises my wife considering that I eat a lot of sugar, especially chocolates, even on Mounjaro.

I had little side effects. The main one was diarrhoea, and even that happened when I ate more food than the drug would let me eat. There has been no change in the kind of food that I eat, but I eat a lot less. My wife and I order fewer dishes in restaurants, and I am able to eat very little of those too. When I travel, I like to and often need to try many different foods and restaurants apart from what comes out of our own kitchen for the catering events. So, I now travel for six days instead of three, because I can't eat that much food in three days.

6

The Chakravyuh: Why It's So Hard to Lose Weight

Putting on weight is often like entering the Chakravyuh, the moving maze of a military formation in the Mahabharata. Very few knew how to get out of it. Many obese patients are like Abhimanyu, who made his way in but didn't know how to exit. If anything, obesity is a progressive disease that often gets worse with time. Everything that looks like an exit turns out to be a dead end.

As stated in earlier chapters, patients taking GLP-1 drugs report disappearance of 'food noise'. It's that voice in the head that seeks food, and craves flavour and crunch all the time. Patients are surprised at their ability to look at their favourite food and leave the table without eating it. It's as if a switch has been turned off, and they're finally finding a way out of the Chakravyuh.

The Chakravyuh: Why It's So Hard to Lose Weight

This patient experience has given us a new understanding of obesity management. It tells us why the standard diet and exercise advice doesn't work for many. It has also highlighted the importance of the brain in the success of GLP-1 medications.

When GLP-1 drugs were first found to be causing weight loss, it was thought to be because they slowed gastric emptying. But it is increasingly clear that the role of the brain is more important. The reduction of appetite is thanks to the GLP-1 receptors in the brain.

Gastric side effects, such as nausea and vomiting, also have to do with the brain. After scientists found the newer GLP-1 drugs were causing significant weight loss, they were able to localize GLP-1 receptors in the brain.

Patients unable to lose weight despite a lot of effort often feel some force inside them is not letting them abstain from food. We can now say that the brain pathway of the GLP-1 hormone has proved this intuition. It seems that people who are unable to lose weight despite making efforts are wired differently. The hunger and craving come not from the stomach but from the brain, which sometimes wants more food than the body needs.

The interaction of the brain hormones with those of the body seems to be a key determinant here. GLP-1 drugs act on the brain via their receptors to produce their beneficial effects on appetite and satiety. American television host

Oprah Winfrey, talking about her experience of losing weight with GLP-1 drugs, has said that she finally understood how thin people stayed thin. It's not that they had more willpower to resist food. They just didn't feel hungry.

This may also explain why many put on weight even after bariatric surgery. The brain still wants to eat more than what the truncated stomach pouch can hold.

At the same time, we did not have today's obesity rates fifty years ago. Our brains could not have changed so rapidly. There's a lot more to why we put on weight and why it is so hard to lose it.

The Obesogenic Environment

'Sacrifice at least one meal a week!' That was not a dietician's advice. That was Prime Minister Lal Bahadur Shastri in 1965, asking the public to cope with India's food shortage in the midst of a war.

Until the late 1960s, we were a 'ship-to-mouth' economy. We waited for the next shipload of foodgrains to arrive from the US as part of an aid programme.

The crisis led to the Green Revolution, in which scientists from the US helped Indian farmers grow high-yield varieties of wheat and rice with improved irrigation, chemical fertilizers and pesticides. There was so much

The Chakravyuh: Why It's So Hard to Lose Weight

wheat and rice around in a few years that India had to shut down theatres and schools to store them.

Today, India is able to provide free foodgrains to 80 crore Indians and still export some. Yet, the Green Revolution has also been a major reason for our obesity epidemic. Refined carbohydrates – wheat, maida and rice – are easy to overeat, lack nutrients as compared to the millets they replaced and cause sugar spikes and insulin resistance.

These high-energy grains, once necessary to feed a hungry nation, are today a leading cause of the obesity crisis. Replacing them with unprocessed grains like millets at home is difficult, but those who are able to do so often see significant weight loss.

Sometimes I get patients wondering why they have put on weight when they hardly eat out and stick to homemade dal–chawal. And while dal is a source of protein, it also contains a significant amount of carbohydrates and is often steeped in ghee or oil. The chawal we consume is often of the highly refined, shiny grain variety. Dal–chawal without enough protein, fibre and vegetables can be a source of carbohydrate-derived calories. A balanced meal needs vegetables, salads and much more protein than most Indians eat as staple 'home food'.

Processed food, easily available everywhere in shiny packets, is invariably heavy in carbohydrates and calories.

It is impossible to get healthy food at airports and railway stations, in school canteens and even in hospital canteens.

Big food companies go to great lengths to hack into your brain's reward systems, giving you crispy, crunchy, sugary and salty snacks you can't resist having. You can't have just one. These are known as hyper-palatable foods. The obesogenic environment we all live in promotes refined carbohydrates over complex ones, sugary desserts over fruits, bread over vegetables and starch over protein.

Obesity prevalence in urban India is much higher than in rural India, and is higher in economically developed states. According to the National Family Health Survey (2019–21), the overall prevalence of abdominal obesity in the country was found to be 40 per cent in women and 12 per cent in men. Five–six out of ten women between the ages of thirty and forty-nine are abdominally obese. In studies on schoolchildren in Delhi, we found such a huge contrast in height and weight between private and government schools that they could well be from different countries. You don't need data to observe that the poor and the working class have far less obesity and diabetes than the affluent. But abdominal obesity is also on the rise in rural areas and is penetrating lower- and middle-socioeconomic sections of society because of a decline in physical activity and an increase in junk food consumption. That alone is proof that the main driver of the obesity epidemic is lifestyle. Urbanization and affluence make us move less and eat more.

I try to explain to my patients that lifestyle modifications is itself a treatment. Only a small proportion of my patients succeed at losing substantial amounts of weight with lifestyle modifications. Of those who do succeed, the majority are unable to prevent it from returning in the long run. Over the years, multiple studies have shown that around 80 per cent people who lose weight gain most of it back within a few years. Half the lost weight returns within two years.

Only five people in the Mahabharata knew how to escape the Chakravyuh. Those who can prevent weight rebound – what do they do right? The ones I have seen achieve this in my clinical practice have generally been younger, and a key factor was that they didn't understand how and why they had put on a lot of weight in the first place. Knowledge helped. Unlike Japan, children are not taught enough about nutrition in our schools. A lot of young people learn what protein, fibre and carbohydrates are only after they start putting on weight. Sometimes I hear back from such young patients who report that my guidance to them about a diet and exercise plan had worked, helping them lose weight or even send their diabetes into remission.

While we consume more calories, the obesogenic environment makes it difficult to lose them. Our cities have become less walkable, lifts are making us not take stairs, cars prevent us from walking, even to the bus or metro stations.

Ironically, progress and development make our environment obesogenic. When a village home gets tap water, the woman no longer walks to the well or burns calories at the hand pump. Packaged foods (such as noodles, chips and biscuits) and bottled sweet beverages have penetrated the rural hinterland. No wonder we are seeing obesity rates rise in the rural areas too.

Indians, particularly those living in large cities and metros, are among the most overworked people in the world, often struggling to find time to have healthy food and exercise. But each one of us must try and modify our lifestyles to fight the obesogenic environment. If nothing else, it will at least prevent further weight gain. The benefits of exercise and a balanced diet go beyond weight management, to aiding cardiovascular health, reducing inflammation and insulin resistance, and building muscle even without weight loss.

I stopped being preachy with my patients about lifestyle modifications long ago. It doesn't work; only adds to the guilt, blame, shame and stress. It is also unfair to be preachy about lifestyle because radical behavioural change is extremely hard. It requires people to forgo their comfort zones and reimagine their lives, routines, work and kitchens.

The Chakravyuh: Why It's So Hard to Lose Weight

For example, often when a woman in India gives birth, she has to look after the child and continue looking after the husband and in-laws, and is also possibly going through postpartum depression. She has no time to look after herself. Preaching lifestyle modifications to her is only going to add to her stress.

If unhealthy food is coming into the house, you will be tempted to eat it. But in families it is hard for one person to say that chips and cookies shouldn't be bought at all because others in the family want them and may not (yet) be struggling to lose weight.

For young male migrants living alone or with flatmates, there may not be the time or willingness to cook, given that cooking in our culture has been the woman's job (though this is changing now). Hiring a cook may not be viable. Eating out and ordering in all the time may become normal. Restaurant food is usually heavy in carbohydrates and full of calorie-rich cooking oil.

It is well known that lack of hydration can come in the way of losing weight. Yet people struggle with behavioural change to even replace their sugar soda with water when having a meal.

People quitting smoking or alcohol find they're eating more food, especially carbs and sugar, to fight their alcohol or nicotine cravings. They put on weight, exchanging one problem for another.

Having sweets used to be something people indulged in on festivals, birthdays and weddings. Today people want *meetha* after every meal. Growing affluence has brought the elites into a hedonistic lifestyle where excess of everything includes excess of calories.

You can try to not give sugar to your child, but it becomes difficult to manage when visiting friends and family offer them candies. It is no surprise that we are seeing an explosion of obesity among children. Children should be taught from an early age how to distinguish between healthy and unhealthy foods, and this should be part of the school curriculum.

Socializing means feasting, and alcohol is a lot of calories too. How do you go to someone's house for tea and say no to that samosa they put before you? How do you go for a dinner party and refuse biryani? 'It's okay, have a bit, you can get back to your diet from tomorrow,' your host will tell you. Tomorrow never comes.

Genes Load the Gun

For thousands of years, India endured frequent famines and periods of food scarcity. There were many reasons for this: erratic monsoons, high population, colonial exploitation, natural disasters, and so on. Indians survived food scarcity by learning to store fat efficiently and burn it in times of need. That is why Indians are genetically more prone to obesity. We are programmed to store fat. This is known as the 'thrifty gene' theory. When a population that's genetically trained to store fat hits an obesogenic environment, you get an obesity epidemic.

While Indians are genetically more prone to obesity, there are individual factors as well. Overweight and obese individuals often wonder why they put on weight so easily and others with similar lifestyles don't. Why can their spouses keep weight from returning but theirs returns with a vengeance? Maybe their hormone–brain axis is wired differently. They may not even realize that they are eating more calories than they burn.

In some affluent Indian families, pregnant and lactating women are encouraged to eat more than necessary, based on the belief that they need to eat for two people. The child born after nine months is now programmed to overeat, and the mother has a hard time losing the weight she put on. This is why we often see women in India unable to lose weight after childbirth. There is data to show that under thirty years of age, Indian men are more likely to be obese than women. Above thirty, it is women.

In a poor family, the woman may be underfed during pregnancy. The child who is born is now programmed to survive on little food. But they grow up in a world full of burgers, pizzas, cakes and sugar sodas, resulting in obesity.

Scientists have identified several genes that make a person more susceptible to obesity and have estimated that the contribution of these inherited genes in making them obese is as high as 40–70 per cent. Obesity-causing genes may dysregulate appetite, affecting signals from fat tissue, gut and other organs to the brain. They may also make a person more susceptible to forming and storing fat cells, regulating how much they move or exercise, and how their body burns calories, both at rest and after eating. These specific genes may contribute to an imbalance between energy intake and expenditure by influencing appetite, fat storage, physical activity, and calorie burning. It is important to point out that genetic predisposition does not inevitably result in obesity. Genes only load the gun. Lifestyle pulls the trigger.

Fighting Against Your Own Body

People making diet-and-exercise efforts to lose weight often find a part of their brains pulling them in the other direction to resist weight loss. The human body is physiologically designed to return to the peak weight it once had. Trying to lose weight is like fighting against your own body. The body comes to settle at a weight range and tries to maintain it. Remember, the body is programmed to save your fat as energy for the next famine. Until then,

The Chakravyuh: Why It's So Hard to Lose Weight

it likes to take the path of least resistance and do what is enjoyable.

When you lose weight, your metabolism slows down, meaning that your body now spends less energy just existing (BMR) than it used to, not least because it has less weight to carry around. The levels of leptin, a hormone that signals fullness, drop. Ghrelin, a hormone that signals hunger, rises. The fat cells shrink but don't go away and are eager to expand again. The brain defends the body against losing more weight. Losing every additional kilo becomes harder.

When the weight returns, like after a crash diet, some people might put on even more weight than they had lost. Then they try a second time. If they had lost 10 kg the first time, this time they are able to lose only 5 kg. With every cycle of weight loss, they experience diminishing returns. Eventually, they are not able to lose any weight at all, no matter how much they try. The crash diets that had once worked so wonderfully don't seem to work at all.

This happens partly because the brain is now inclined to make your body store more fat for the next time you go on a diet, anticipating a need to prepare for the next famine even harder. The depleting muscle mass with every weight-loss cycle slows down your ability to lose weight in future. Yo-yo dieting causes muscle loss, and in the absence of strength training, makes such patients even more prone to weight gain.

Recent studies in mice show that there are changes in the structure of DNA within fat cells, which also makes it hard to keep weight off after you have lost it. These DNA alterations change how fat cells store and burn fat and the changes stay even after weight loss.

In the previous chapter, we explained how obesity causes insulin resistance, in which insulin has a harder time getting your glucose into the blood cells. Insulin resistance also causes cellular alterations that impede correct sensing of a body's energy balance. Similarly, fat deposits in the liver come in the way of it doing its job of metabolism, digestion and blood purification. In these ways, obesity becomes self-perpetuating, a vicious cycle – a Chakravyuh.

Mental Health

As discussed previously, stress, depression and anxiety are often behind weight gain. Sometimes people put on weight during periods of stress or depression and then struggle forever to lose it. We often hear terms like 'stress eating' or 'comfort eating'. The reciprocal link between depression and obesity is well-established. Some people have chronic anxiety leading to overeating and weight gain.

Stress makes the body release a hormone called cortisol that promotes fat accumulation. As the body feels threatened, it resorts to preparing for future adversities by increasing fat storage. Sometimes I see patients who are doing everything right but are unable to lose weight because of stress. Long-term chronic stress indirectly causes insulin resistance, making it hard to lose weight.

Stress also increases levels of ghrelin, the hunger hormone, making you want to eat more carbohydrates and sugar that feel comforting. Depression makes you less sensitive to dopamine, a hormone that regulates your sense of reward and motivation. The depressed brain needs more reward, and what can be more rewarding than food?

Mental-health issues come in the way of lifestyle modifications. People often eat food as a defence mechanism, as it makes them feel secure. Low motivation doesn't help in sticking to an exercise regimen. Patients struggling to lose weight because of mental-health issues should see a psychologist or psychiatrist. Sadly, the stigma associated with depression doesn't allow many to make that appointment.

Some people have binge-eating disorder, in which they frequently overeat, unable to control their appetite, and often feel distressed after eating. When someone says they can't lose weight because they're 'foodies', it is possible that they have this disorder. Similarly, attention-deficit hyperactivity disorder (ADHD) leads to greater impulsive eating. These conditions often go undiagnosed as patients don't see the importance of psychologists and psychiatrists in treating obesity.

Several studies have shown that fat-shaming does not help obese individuals lose weight. On the contrary, the more a person perceives being discriminated against because of excess weight, the more weight they seem to put on in the long run. The primary cause is that fat-shaming, perceived discrimination and negative self-image add to stress, depression and anxiety. Casually commenting on people's weight and giving unsolicited advice to friends on the need to lose weight does more harm than good.

Sleep

Sleep is the foundation of good health and weight management. Poor quantity and quality of sleep – for whatever reason – increases your hunger levels. This is because, once again, those three hormones are disrupted: leptin, ghrelin and cortisol. The lack of restful sleep makes you fatigued the next day, and the fatigue doesn't let you exercise.

Studies have shown that people who sleep late, work night shifts or eat late at night tend to put on more weight and have higher blood sugar levels. Regulating hunger, satiety and stress hormones requires following the circadian rhythm: early to bed, early to rise.

An often-underdiagnosed condition is obstructive sleep apnoea, without addressing which it is extremely difficult to lose weight. Obese patients who wake up with a headache or snore a lot should take a sleep test, and if diagnosed with sleep apnoea, must use a CPAP machine at night. Fat deposits in the upper airway or around the neck obstruct normal breathing during sleep, thus preventing them from getting deep sleep.

Like many aspects of obesity, this is a vicious cycle – poor sleep causes weight gain, and weight gain further worsens sleep quality. Mental-health conditions also disrupt sleep, as do screens and lack of exercise. Some have chronic insomnia. If patients are unable to improve their sleep quality despite making efforts, they should see a sleep specialist.

Endocrine Disruptors

Many of the conveniences of modern life carry hidden chemicals that cause obesity. These include plastic containers, cosmetics and food packaging. The endocrine-disrupting chemicals (EDCs) in these interfere with the body's hormonal system, altering metabolism, fat storage and appetite regulation. They affect hormones, such as insulin, thyroid, leptin and cortisol, leading to disrupted metabolism. Bisphenol A (BPA), phthalates and persistent organic pollutants (POPs) are common obesogenic chemicals that alter how the body processes energy. Bisphenol A, found in plastic food containers and canned food linings, mimics oestrogen, which can increase fat accumulation.

Some endocrine disruptors promote fat storage by increasing the size and number of fat cells. Phthalates, found in plastics and personal care products, are linked to increased abdominal fat. Endocrine-disrupting chemicals also impair adiponectin, a hormone responsible for breaking down fat, making it easier for the body to store excess weight.

Some EDCs disrupt hunger and satiety hormones like leptin and ghrelin, leading to increased cravings and overeating. Pesticides and flame retardants used for fireproofing also contribute to insulin resistance, making it harder for the body to regulate blood sugar and increasing fat accumulation.

Gut Microbiome

The gut microbiome is a universe of bacteria, viruses, fungi and other microorganisms living in our digestive tract. The composition of the gut microbiome can have far-reaching consequences on our health. An imbalance in the microbial community can lead to inflammation and metabolic disturbances, both of which are linked to obesity.

Some studies suggest that certain gut bacteria can extract more calories from the same amount of food. People with an abundance of such bacteria might put on more weight in the same food as compared to someone who has less of such bacteria.

A healthy gut lining prevents harmful substances from entering the bloodstream. When dysbiosis occurs, it can compromise this barrier, leading to a 'leaky gut', adding to metabolic dysfunction and chronic inflammation.

The gut microbiome can also affect the production of hormones related to hunger and satiety, including GLP-1. Additionally, there is growing evidence that the gut microbiome may affect mood and stress responses, which in turn can influence eating habits and weight management.

The composition of the gut microbiome can make some people more prone to obesity, but a poor diet also makes it a vicious cycle, whereby the obesity-causing bacteria increase in number. Even after weight loss, the gut microbiome may remain biased towards weight regain. Eating a varied diet, including a variety of fruits and vegetables, can help address this.

There is emerging evidence in studies that GLP-1 drugs alter the gut microbiome to increase the quantity of beneficial bacteria.

Ageing

Ageing itself causes weight gain and makes it harder to lose weight. If a person keeps eating the same food and maintains the same level of physical activity all their lives, they might still gain weight.

As we grow older, maintaining a healthy weight becomes more challenging due to slowing metabolism, hormonal shifts, muscle loss and lifestyle changes. These factors contribute to an increased tendency to gain fat, particularly around the abdomen. The pot belly has traditionally been associated with middle age.

For this reason, we need to eat less and exercise more with age. Often, we see the opposite. Ageing causes muscle loss, a condition known as sarcopenia, which reduces BMR, the calories we burn for normal body functions. Without reducing calorie intake, this leads to accumulation of fat. Sometimes it is not so much weight gain as only redistribution of fat due to sarcopenia. Additionally, since muscle is metabolically active, its loss leads to fewer calories burnt at rest, making weight gain more likely. Furthermore, ageing often results in reduced physical activity, either due to joint pain or mobility issues or just a more sedentary lifestyle. This further contributes to muscle loss and fat gain.

Hormonal fluctuations also play a major role in age-related weight gain. Among men, testosterone levels decline with age, leading to muscle loss and increased fat accumulation, especially in the abdominal area. Since muscles burn more calories than fat, muscle loss further reduces metabolic rate, making weight gain more likely.

In women, menopause leads to a drop in oestrogen levels, which causes fat redistribution from the hips and thighs to the abdomen. This shift in fat storage increases the risk of central obesity, which is linked to metabolic diseases.

Ageing also comes with sleep disturbances, and mobility issues like joint pain, reducing physical activity.

Diseases that May Cause Obesity

Some medical conditions also cause weight gain.

Some people have chronically high levels of cortisol, a condition known as Cushing's syndrome. In such cases, we have to treat the source of cortisol – the adrenal or pituitary gland – to provide relief from obesity and other symptoms.

Among women, PCOS can aggravate weight gain. It is a bit of a chicken-and-egg story: PCOS can be caused by weight gain in the first place.

Hypothyroidism has a minor impact on weight gain as it slows down metabolism. Typical weight gain in overt hypothyroidism is 2–4 kg.

Insulin resistance eventually gives way to diabetes, which makes it doubly hard to lose weight for many reasons. Emerging studies suggest that people with diabetes, on average, lose about half the weight on GLP-1 drugs as compared to those without diabetes.

Medicines that May Increase Weight

Weight gain is a common side effect of many medications. Some medicines alter the body's natural processes, leading to increased fat accumulation, fluid retention or changes in appetite. Corticosteroids (prednisone, dexamethasone), prescribed for inflammatory and immunological conditions, can cause the body to retain water, redistribute fat to areas like the face and abdomen, and cause weight gain by increasing appetite.

Some antidepressants affect neurotransmitters like serotonin and histamine, which can enhance cravings for carbohydrates and lead to excessive calorie intake. Similarly, some antipsychotic drugs like olanzapine and risperidone disrupt the body's ability to regulate hunger, causing significant weight gain.

Insulin and sulphonylureas, used for diabetes, encourage fat storage and can cause weight gain if not carefully balanced with diet and exercise. They also contribute to weight gain by producing low blood glucose and, hence, increasing appetite. Pioglitazone, another anti-diabetes medication, leads to significant fat increase and weight gain.

Some medications also lead to fluid retention and bloating, contributing to weight gain that is not necessarily due to fat accumulation. Hormonal medications, including certain birth control pills and hormone replacement therapies, can lead to water retention and changes in body composition.

The good news is, no matter what the reason for your obesity, GLP-1 drugs seem to work. In the end, the calorie deficit maths reigns supreme. If you consume less calories than you burn, you will lose weight. GLP-1 drugs help you with reducing consumption. They are helping people come out of the Chakravyuh of obesity by solving one part of the puzzle: helping them eat less. It will still remain important to eat right and exercise consistently for long-term health outcomes.

Takeaway

Many people who lose weight through diet and exercise find that it returns, sometimes with a vengeance. There are multiple reasons why people put on weight and find it hard to lose it sustainably. GLP-1 drugs are showing us that people who are unable to lose weight with diet and exercise may well have their brains wired differently. A multitude of reasons prevent people from losing weight, from genetic predisposition to medications.

PATENT STORY

RAMONA, 50

My HbA1c used to hover around 6.5, borderline diabetes. One day, when I found out it had reached 6.9, I decided to try Mounjaro. With the guidance of Dr Mithal, I started the drug. I have lost 10 kg, and I am now in the pre-diabetes range.

I have taken to diet and exercise many times, but the lost weight would inevitably return. I have long been a healthy eater. I once went to a nutritionist and told her what my diet was. She had nothing to add or subtract. I had it all figured out. But my problem was portion control. A kind of greed would overcome me.

With Mounjaro, the loss of appetite takes care of that problem. When I used to go on a diet, I would think all day about what I had to eat and how much, and how to stay disciplined. With Mounjaro, I don't have to think about food. The dieting is painless. The medicine ensures I don't overeat even if the food tastes very good.

On Mounjaro, one can also lose weight without exercise, but I have consciously maintained a regular exercise regimen. The weight loss has given me a psychological high that keeps me motivated.

The Chakravyuh: Why It's So Hard to Lose Weight

The starting dose didn't do much for me. I had mild nausea, minor weight loss and better sugar control. But 5 mg felt powerful. I had enough nausea that I had to take a pill for it on the first day or two. This happens even now every time I take the weekly injection regardless of the dose. There is mild nausea for a day or two, and then it goes away. Every time I start a new dose, I also have an upset stomach for a few days.

My HbA1c is around 6. I don't check my sugar often as I think it is in the safe range now.

When I reached the 12.5 mg dose, I also had some vomiting and a lot of diarrhoea, so I went back to 10 mg. After being on 10 mg for four months, I started on 12.5 mg again and this time, I have no side effects, no nausea and the hunger has returned. I have gained back 2 kg. Maybe it's a faulty pen. I'm hoping this is just a bad patch.

7

The Happy Side Effects

Research into the sugar-lowering powers of incretin hormones led to the discovery of GLP-1 drugs. The added bonus of weight loss was serendipity.

There seem to be many happy side effects of GLP-1 drugs. Of course, many of them are not because of the drugs themselves but because of weight loss. When you lose weight – whether through diet and exercise, bariatric surgery, or GLP-1 drugs – your knee pain and inflammation will reduce, heart health will improve, and so on.

Yet it seems that GLP-1 drugs are directly improving health outcomes as well, apart from the benefits that accrue by reducing blood sugar and hunger. Dr. Daniel Drucker, one of the scientists who discovered the GLP-1 hormone, conducted an experiment on mice with systemic inflammation. When treated with GLP-1 drugs, the inflammation decreased. However, if the drug was blocked from reaching the brain, the inflammation did not reduce. **This suggests that the brain plays a critical role in inflammation, and that reducing it may be directly mediated through the brain and not just indirectly due to weight loss.**

GLP-1 receptors – the switches activated by the drug – are found in the heart, liver, kidneys, pancreas, stomach, intestines and brain. As with many hormones, GLP-1's effects may not be limited to hunger and satiety alone but may also have multiple other functions. The full range of benefits these drugs can have in treating various diseases is still being discovered.

In October 2018, Novo Nordisk, the company that holds the patent for semaglutide, began a trial to study the impact of the drug on the cardiovascular health of people who had heart disease and were overweight or obese but did not have diabetes. They enrolled over 17,000 people from diverse backgrounds. Their mean BMI was 33, and nobody was less than BMI 27. They were divided into two similar groups. One was given semaglutide (Wegovy) and the other was given a placebo.

As the trial progressed, Covid-19 struck. Both groups saw similar rates of infection. Among the 184 who died of Covid-19, 78 had been taking semaglutide and 106 were on placebo. The difference is significant enough to suggest that the drug helped save some lives.

In the trial, some died of reasons other than the pandemic. After accounting for all causes of death, those taking the drug saw 19 per cent less fatality.

No, this does not mean that GLP-1 drugs can be a treatment for Covid-19. What it does show is that the drug is improving overall health through weight loss and reduced inflammation. It confirms what we know about obesity: It's a disease.

Did some of those patients survive the pandemic only because weight loss improved their overall health, or also because the drug reduced their inflammation levels, or were there more reasons? This is an open question because scientists are still discovering the full range of what GLP-1 drugs do inside the body. Their action on various diseases could help understand the disease better, perhaps aiding the discovery of new specific drugs and treatments for those diseases. GLP-1 drugs themselves could, some day, be prescribed for many of those conditions.

A Growing List

It is important to note that research is ongoing and incomplete. Patients should not self-medicate. Even if GLP-1 drugs are approved by the US FDA or other regulators for some of these conditions, they must be used only under medical supervision.

Here are some medical conditions in which GLP-1 drugs have been found to be helpful so far.

Heart Disease

In March 2024, the US FDA approved Wegovy (semaglutide, same as Ozempic) for patients who had heart disease along with obesity or were overweight even if they did not have diabetes. This followed a large trial called SELECT (the same trial that showed the Covid-19 effect fortuitously), which had 17,600 patients enrolled in two groups. In the placebo group, 8 per cent participants saw major adverse cardiovascular events (MACEs), such as heart attack, stroke or cardiovascular death. In the group taking semaglutide, the incidence was 6.5 per cent. That's a nearly 20 per cent reduction in risk. While this trial used weekly injectable semaglutide, the more recent SOUL trial, involving almost 10,000 participants, used oral semaglutide (Rybelsus) and showed a reduction in MACE of 14 per cent. Statins remain the main drug for people with heart disease, but these results demonstrate the role of semaglutide in prevention of heart disease on top of statin therapy.

Tirzepatide (GIP + GLP-1) has also been shown to reduce cardiovascular risk. In an international trial of 713 adults in nine countries, including the US, called the SUMMIT trial, participants with heart failure taking tirzepatide for two years had significantly improved cardiovascular health and reduced progression of heart failure.

An analysis of thirteen GLP-1 drug trials comprising more than 80,000 patients showed significant reductions in MACE, overall and cardiovascular mortality, stroke, and need for coronary procedures like angioplasty and surgery, regardless of the presence of diabetes. The benefits could not be explained by weight loss alone.

These trials have led to guidelines that all people with diabetes and/or obesity who either suffer from or are at risk of heart disease should be treated with GLP-1 drugs. However, since people with diabetes and/or obesity are at higher risk of heart attack and stroke anyway, it is prudent to consider the prescription of these drugs in most people with diabetes even if they have no evidence of heart disease.

Chronic Kidney Disease

In January 2025, the US FDA approved the use of semaglutide in patients who have both diabetes and kidney disease. Our kidneys filter out toxins from the body and pass them through the urine. Their ability to do so starts declining in patients with diabetes. The FLOW trial showed that for patients with both type 2 diabetes and chronic kidney disease, taking semaglutide lowered the risk of complications (dialysis, need for transplant) by 24 per cent. It also slowed down the decline of their kidney function.

Moreover, in a post hoc analysis of the SURPASS-4 randomized clinical trial, tirzepatide decreased protein excretion, slowed decline in kidney function and reduced death due to kidney causes in patients with type 2 diabetes.

Cancer

Since obesity raises the risk of some types of cancer, it is not surprising that studies have started finding a reduced incidence of cancer among those taking GLP-1 drugs. This is similar to the reduced risk of cancer seen among those who have undergone bariatric surgery. Obesity-related cancers are concentrated around the metabolic organs and, among women, around the reproductive organs as well. An observational study of 1.65 million patients in the US found a reduced risk of ten types of obesity-related cancers among diabetes patients taking GLP-1 drugs as compared to those on insulin. Another study found the risk of 13 types of cancer reduced by 22 per cent in those who underwent bariatric surgery and by 39 per cent among those who took GLP-1 drugs.

Liver Disease

Metabolic dysfunction-associated steatotic liver disease, popularly known as fatty liver disease, is a common result of obesity. In its advanced form it can lead to MASH, or metabolic dysfunction-associated steatohepatitis, and eventually to liver cirrhosis and liver cancer, which can be fatal (as discussed in Chapter 5). GLP-1 drugs have been shown to be effective in reducing body weight, liver injury indices and liver fat content. Several studies also suggest that these drugs are able to promote the resolution of steatohepatitis in some patients with MASH and possibly reduce the progression of hepatic fibrosis. The mechanism is likely through both metabolic improvements and direct reduction in inflammation. This is not surprising given the direct link between obesity and fatty liver disease. However, GLP-1 drugs have so far not been approved specifically for these liver conditions. Additional benefits for liver health apart from weight loss and sugar control are expected from double (tirzepatide, survodutide) and triple agonists (retatrutide), but results from specific human clinical trials are awaited.

Alzheimer's Disease

Alzheimer's is a progressive neuro-degenerative disorder that affects memory, thinking and behaviour. It is the leading cause of dementia. Chronic inflammation often underlies Alzheimer's. Research in rodents has shown that GLP-1 drugs can improve features of Alzheimer's, but human trials are ongoing. Observational data among people taking GLP-1 drugs has shown a lower risk of Alzheimer's. People with type 2 diabetes have an increased risk of dementia. Randomized trials and observational studies have found that GLP-1 drugs reduce the incidence of dementia in people with diabetes.

This may partly be because improvement in obesity and diabetes reduces the risk of dementia, but likely also because GLP-1 drugs may reduce inflammation in the brain.

Research on Parkinson's has also been promising but has been focused chiefly on the very first GLP-1 drug, exenatide.

Hypertension

GLP-1 drugs have been shown to lower blood pressure in several trials. Studies involving the older GLP-1 drugs, liraglutide and dulaglutide, showed a decline in blood pressure. The SUSTAIN and PIONEER trials showed a decline in systolic blood pressure with semaglutide.

The SURMOUNT-1 trial found that patients taking tirzepatide (Mounjaro, Zepbound) for thirty-six weeks had significantly lower blood pressure, corresponding to weight loss. The change, measured through twenty-four-hour blood pressure monitors, was as significant as that achieved by blood pressure medications.

Overall reduction in blood pressure with GLP-1 drugs is to the tune of 2–4 mmHg. While weight reduction is an important reason for this decline in blood pressure, a direct action of the drugs on the blood vessels via the GLP-1 receptors is also possible. The mild increase in urine output produced by these drugs might also be a factor in reducing blood pressure.

Rheumatoid Arthritis

Preclinical studies suggest GLP-1 drugs can directly reduce the severity of rheumatoid arthritis. While human trials are awaited, a number of rheumatoid arthritis patients taking GLP-1 drugs have reported remarkable improvement. After Dr Daniel Drucker released his study on the link between GLP-1 and inflammation, a woman sent him photos of her hands, taken before and after starting tirzepatide (Zepbound) for weight loss. The photos showed her swelling disappearing after taking the drug. She told *The New York Times* that her joint pain from rheumatoid arthritis went away within a few days of starting the drug, indicating a reduction in inflammation independent of weight loss. Such anecdotal evidence is mounting.

Knee Osteoarthritis

A trial found that overweight or obese patients who also had knee osteoarthritis, saw their knee pain reduced by almost half after taking semaglutide (Ozempic). Knee arthritis is caused mainly by the wearing down of knee cartilage, a process aggravated in overweight and obese patients due to the mechanical effect of having to carry excess weight. But there is also inflammation beyond cartilage damage, and the ability of GLP-1 drugs to bring down inflammation directly is also suspected to be a factor in reducing pain.

Psoriasis

This is an autoimmune skin disorder often accompanied by metabolic disorders. GLP-1 drugs have been found in small studies to significantly reduce the severity of psoriasis even before significant weight loss, indicating direct anti-inflammatory action.

PCOS

Insulin resistance and excess weight trigger hormonal imbalances in women that may cause PCOS. The condition may cause acne, excess body hair, high testosterone levels, irregular periods and infertility. Weight loss often makes it go away. Weight loss and reduction in insulin sensitivity are the main drivers of improvement in PCOS among women taking GLP-1 drugs.

Infertility

There have been several anecdotal reports of women from across the world getting pregnant after taking GLP-1 drugs even though they had been told they would not be able to conceive for some reason, PCOS being only one of them. These surprise pregnancies are mostly attributed to improvement in overall metabolic health due to weight loss.

There have also been reports of women on GLP-1 drugs getting pregnant despite taking birth control pills. Eli Lilly, the company that makes Mounjaro, has advised women taking these drugs to switch to non-oral contraceptives or consult their doctor to switch to a different birth control pill. It is speculated that birth control pills may not be properly absorbed into the bloodstream during the initial phase of a new or higher dose of the drug, possibly due to reduced appetite.

Alcoholism and Reward System Disorders

Many patients taking GLP-1 drugs report a significant drop in their desire to drink alcohol. This is beginning to be confirmed in trials. A study published in February 2025 found that among patients taking semaglutide, alcohol consumption dropped by 30 per cent. Some people taking GLP-1 drugs say they just don't feel like drinking alcohol anymore, while some who were binge drinkers are now able to drink in moderation. This seems to be similar to what the drugs do to their food intake. However, animal studies have shown that these drugs may also inhibit the release of alcohol-related dopamine. Researchers are trying to investigate if these drugs can also help treat other reward system disorders such as smoking and substance abuse. Studies based on patient records in hospitals are showing a significant reduction in opioid use disorder as well as alcoholism. As of now, it is not clear if these drugs could help treat alcoholism among those who are not overweight or obese.

Sleep Apnoea

The US FDA has approved tirzepatide (Mounjaro) in patients who are obese and have sleep apnoea after a trial found a reduction in the severity of the disease. This was related directly to weight loss. Patients with sleep apnoea should not substitute CPAP therapy with GLP-1 drugs but use them together. After reaching the target weight, you may review with your doctor if it is good to discontinue CPAP therapy.

Asthma

Studies show a reduction in the severity of asthma among overweight and obese patients with the use of GLP-1 drugs. The improvement is said to be not only because of weight loss but also reduced airway inflammation. The lungs also have GLP-1 receptors, raising the possibility of direct improvement in lung health irrespective of weight loss.

GLP-1 as an Anti-Ageing Drug

Barely a week goes by in which we don't discover some new positive effect of GLP-1 drugs. These discoveries, made easier by artificial intelligence (AI) scanning through patient records in no time, are helping scientists understand many diseases better and could lead to advancements in healthcare beyond the mere administration of GLP-1 drugs.

If these drugs can do so much, it makes us wonder if we have finally found an anti-ageing potion. Apart from increasing lifespan by reducing the burden of metabolic diseases, can GLP-1 drugs directly increase longevity?

According to Dr Daniel Drucker, organs with GLP-1 receptors 'seem to allow cells to be maintained in a healthier state and to be less susceptible to death'.

Reducing inflammation independent of weight loss can help improve overall health outcomes even beyond the organs with GLP-1 receptors. Chronic inflammation damages tissues and contributes to cancer and cardiovascular, neuro-degenerative and autoimmune diseases.

How do these drugs, or the GLP-1 hormone, reduce inflammation even where there are no GLP-1 receptors? The answer lies in the human body's central processing unit, the brain. The effect on inflammation seems to also be mediated through the brain. This raises the possibility that GLP-1 drugs could have an anti-ageing effect, apart from the benefits of treating obesity and diabetes.

Takeaway

GLP-1 drugs were developed for diabetes and found to be good for weight loss. But they may be doing a lot more beyond sugar control and weight management. By directly reducing inflammation and regulating hormone signalling with the brain, they may have a multitude of health benefits. Research on these benefits of GLP-1 drugs is progressing at a hectic pace.

PATIENT STORY

MANSHA BHATIA, 26

A knee injury in 2016 had me walking with crutches for eight months. The weight I gained in those months refused to go away for years. I went on crash diets, balanced diets, sometimes barely eating anything all day, and I did a lot of exercise. Yet the weight just wouldn't go away. Going to the gym sometimes made me put on even more weight. Weight gain gave me PCOS, and the PCOS seemed to hinder my efforts to lose weight.

I had reached a BMI of 34 and wanted to try a GLP-1 drug because nothing else would work. Friends, family and the Internet scared me a lot about the side effects. I went to Dr Mithal and discussed the side effects with him, and soon, I started Mounjaro 2.5 mg. Dr Mithal had prepared me for the side effects that came – nausea, diarrhoea, headaches – but they were never so bad that they came in the way of daily life.

I have lost 18 kg in eight months and my PCOS has completely gone away. My back pain, knee pain and breathlessness have also disappeared. At a BMI of 34, I also had acid reflux, often felt lethargic and it didn't feel good

> *looking at myself in the mirror. I feel a lot better now. My blood reports look a lot better on various counts.*
>
> *I want to be 58 kg but Dr Mithal says 65 kg is fine and I should now be on a maintenance dose. In fact, after two months on 10 mg, when I still had some gastric side effects, he lowered my dose to 7.5 mg. Lowering the dose did not make me put on the weight I had lost. I'm still losing some weight, but slowly.*
>
> *There were days on Mounjaro when I couldn't eat anything all day but as I got used to a new dose, I was able to eat just about the amount food that I needed. My food habits have become healthier. I stick to home food and exercise consistently, both cardio and strength training.*

8

A Revolution in Diabetes Management

In the fifth century BCE, the Indian physician Sushruta noticed that ants were attracted to some people's urine, leading him to discover that such people had a condition that caused their urine to be sweet and sticky. He named the disease *madhumeha* or honey-like urine. He also found that those with this disease were primarily the rich classes, and they consumed excessive rice, cereals and sweets. Today, we call this type 2 diabetes or 'diabetes mellitus'. The word 'diabetes' comes from ancient Greece, and means *siphon* or 'to pass through', a reference to excessive urination the condition causes. *Mellitus* is Latin for 'honey-sweet'.

Diabetes is a chronic condition in which the body either doesn't produce enough insulin, or is unable to use it well. The hormone insulin helps glucose enter the cells and thus provides energy to the body. If insulin is deficient or ineffective, glucose can't enter the cells. Left to circulate in the blood, high glucose levels start harming the body and its organs.

There are two types of diabetes, type 1 and type 2. Type 1 is usually an autoimmune disorder in which the pancreas cannot produce insulin. Classically, type 1 was thought to occur only in children, have an acute onset and had to be treated only with insulin. While insulin treatment still remains mandatory for type 1, we now see many variants of the condition. For example, it can occur in adults and the onset can be slow.

GLP-1 drugs are not for type 1 diabetes unless a type 1 patient has put on a lot of weight and their doctor decides to calibrate their insulin and GLP-1 drugs carefully. For type 2, however, GLP-1 drugs have been a revolution.

Around 90 per cent of people with diabetes have type 2, which is usually accompanied by insulin resistance. It is often the initial defect in type 2 diabetes. As mentioned in Chapter 5, the pancreas makes insulin, but there is resistance to insulin action at the cellular level. As a result, insulin action on the cell is incomplete and ineffective. Insulin is the key that opens the lock for glucose to enter the cells to provide them energy. If the lock is rusted, the key won't turn easily, the door won't open and glucose will continue accumulating in the bloodstream instead of going where it is needed.

Trying to break the rusty lock on the door of the cell and control the rising levels of glucose in the blood, the pancreas ramps up the production of insulin. At some point, it can't keep up and the pancreatic function starts declining. The moment the pancreas starts giving up is when the patient gets elevated blood glucose or type 2 diabetes. By this time, the patient has already lost 50 per cent of their pancreatic function.

There are many kinds of type 2 diabetes patients. We call them clusters. There are those whose predominant issue is insulin deficiency, those who predominantly have insulin resistance, those with both, and some who are elderly with mild diabetes as pancreatic function starts declining with age. Yet it is not just insulin resistance that may cause diabetes (henceforth, when we say 'diabetes', we imply type 2). There may be some other causes, too.

One is the incretin defect. Incretin hormones GLP-1 and GIP are secreted naturally in the gut in response to food. It is possible that in some people there may not be enough production of the incretin hormones. The GLP-1 hormone stimulates the production of insulin, which lowers blood glucose, and suppresses glucagon. Glucagon is a hormone that raises glucose, countering the action of insulin. GLP-1 acts to balance these two.

This is why the effort to create GLP-1 drugs was all about controlling diabetes. Weight loss, and the other hormone actions, were discovered later as a by-product.

A Revolution in Diabetes Management

The Diabetes Epidemic in India

A study published in 2023 by the Indian Council of Medical Research and India Diabetes (ICMR-INDIAB) found that 11.3 per cent of India's adult population has diabetes, and another 15.3 per cent has pre-diabetes, in which glucose levels are higher than normal but not high enough to be categorized as diabetes.

Many Indians don't find it necessary to get a blood test, and as a result, at least 50 per cent of those with diabetes are unaware that they have the condition. One can have diabetes for five to ten years without showing any symptoms. There may be some fatigue, but people often explain it away. Who doesn't feel a bit tired these days?

Screening for diabetes is very important. Conventional wisdom used to be that everyone above forty must get screened annually for diabetes. Nowadays, in India, we advise people to start doing so after twenty-five years of age. There is a sharp increase in diabetes incidence after people reach twenty-five.

What explains this explosion of diabetes? Our genes haven't changed. It starts with nutrition and lifestyle. If you move from villages to small towns, the prevalence of diabetes roughly doubles. If you go from small towns to metros, it doubles again. The ICMR-INDIAB study found the incidence of diabetes is the highest in urban areas like Delhi, Goa and Chandigarh. Jharkhand has a huge urban–rural gap in diabetes. In a more developed state like Kerala, the urban–rural gap has disappeared.

Changes in our diet, exercise patterns, endocrine disruptors like microplastics, high levels of stress, poor sleep and air pollution are some of the reasons fuelling the diabetes epidemic. If this sounds like the factors behind the obesity epidemic we discussed in Chapter 6, it is because obesity and diabetes go together. **It is uncommon to see patients with type 2 diabetes who aren't also overweight or obese.** Even if some of them appear lean, they tend to have high visceral fat. Some might think this correlation is well known, but you'll be surprised to see that many people with diabetes who come to me don't know the link. Sometimes, I struggle to explain to them that they need to lose weight even if medicines have brought their sugar levels under control. Without weight management, their diabetes is bound to worsen again with time, requiring progressively more medication and causing other health complications.

Some people become very obese but do not develop diabetes. Genetic reasons explain this phenomenon. Even such a person will have insulin resistance, but the pancreas holds up against the onslaught of glucose, producing enough insulin to prevent diabetes. Similarly, some people might develop diabetes with just a little bit of extra weight, indicating insulin deficiency and not just resistance.

Sometimes what may look like just a little extra weight might be years of visceral fat, the most harmful kind.

In obese patients, an often-underdiagnosed contributor to diabetes is poor sleep. Poor quality and quantity of sleep raises stress levels, contributing to weight gain and, thus, insulin resistance. A study in China found that diabetes levels rise in cities with bright lights at night. Similarly, night-shift workers are at a higher risk of diabetes. The circadian rhythm, the body's natural clock, helps regulate various metabolic hormones, including insulin.

Sleep apnoea causes hypoxia – low blood oxygen levels – which also leads to insulin resistance. This happens when fat deposits around the neck and the tongue prevent the patient from breathing freely in sleep, leading to snoring and airway blockage. Without a CPAP machine that keeps the airways open and allows the patient to breathe freely in sleep, such patients will find it hard to bring down their blood sugar levels and lose weight.

Modern development and urbanization have also contributed to the diabetes epidemic in other ways. Air pollution in the form of particulate matter as small as 2.5 micrometres (PM 2.5) can enter the bloodstream through the lungs. It excites inflammation in the pancreas and even in the adipose tissue. This suppresses insulin secretion and also increases resistance to the insulin being produced.

The Global Burden of Disease assessment estimates that 20 per cent of global type 2 diabetes cases are related to chronic exposure to PM 2.5. With 99 per cent of the global population residing in areas where air pollution levels are above current WHO air quality guidelines, this is a major concern. Another study published in the *British Medical Journal* in 2023 followed a cohort of 12,000 men and women in Delhi and Chennai from 2010 to 2017. The study found that even one month of exposure to PM 2.5 raised blood sugar levels. Exposure for a year raised the risk of diabetes, as well as hypertension. This is apart from other health conditions, such as lung diseases, whose link to air pollution is more obvious.

It's Complicated

One of the ways diabetes is diagnosed is through a blood test called HbA1c, which measures average blood sugar levels over the last two-three months. An HbA1c of 5.6 per cent or less is normal; between 5.7 per cent and 6.4 per cent indicates pre-diabetes. If the HbA1c is at 6.5 per cent or above, it is diabetes.

In the early stages of diabetes, lifestyle changes and weight loss can help with the remission of the disease. Research has shown that for every 1 percentage point decrease in body weight, the chances of complete remission increase by 2 per cent. In one study called the DiRECT trial, 36 per cent participants with diabetes who lost an average of 7.6 kg in two years were able to achieve remission. After another three years, 34 per cent participants who continued weight loss intervention were able to keep diabetes in remission.

People often use the term 'reversal' for diabetes, but remission is more accurate. Reversal implies permanence. Sometimes, a patient may improve their sugar levels such that it is technically not in the diabetes range and think they have 'reversed' diabetes, but after putting on some weight again, their HbA1c may be back in the diabetic range.

The distinction between pre-diabetes and diabetes is not based on different levels of insulin or insulin resistance but on the risk of complications. Since high blood sugar levels can cause numerous health issues, the entire focus is on 'controlling' sugar levels to prevent these complications.

The focus of research and treatment on pre-diabetes is to prevent it from progressing to diabetes. However, recent studies show a greater risk of health complications, especially heart disease, even in the pre-diabetes stage. People with pre-diabetes would do well to not see it only as a warning for diabetes but as a disease by itself. The primary treatment for pre-diabetes is weight loss.

Among the most common complications of diabetes is neuropathy, in which nerve damage causes tingling and pain in hands and feet, sometimes even in internal organs.

Unchecked diabetes can also damage the retina, a condition called diabetic retinopathy, resulting in vision loss and even blindness. Kidney damage is often seen in advanced diabetes, which can progress to kidney failure. Dialysis and transplant are the ultimate treatment options. Diabetes is also one of the factors in raising the risk matrix of cardiovascular disease. Heart attacks account for more than 70 per cent of diabetes-related deaths. Peripheral artery disease narrows the blood vessels in the legs, leading to poor circulation, pain and risk of amputation. Wounds often don't heal easily in diabetes. Sometimes, diabetic foot ulcers can raise the risk of the infection spreading, making amputations necessary.

Diabetes increases the incidence of hearing loss, erectile dysfunction, Alzheimer's, dementia and gastroparesis. It also increases the susceptibility to bacterial and fungal infections due to weakened immunity.

The goal of diabetes treatment is to prevent these complications. People with diabetes can and do lead happy, everyday lives by keeping their sugar levels under control. The longer a patient has had diabetes, the greater the chances of complications. Then there is genetic risk. We see entire families where diabetes has often led to a particular complication, such as, say, kidney disease.

These complications are apart from the diseases caused by obesity itself, as explained in Chapter 5. A patient with obesity and diabetes also often has hypertension and heart disease. Endocrinologists have an ABCD approach to reduce the overall risk of complications and increase life expectancy. A stands for A1c (HbA1c), underlining the importance of good sugar control. B stands for blood pressure, usually managed with medication. C is for cholesterol (LDL cholesterol), where statins are almost always needed to prevent heart attacks. These A, B and C are partners in crime, often working together to cause complications.

The targets for each of these have to be individualized, depending on the patient's age and accompanying comorbidities. Still, a general rule of thumb is to aim for an HbA1c less than 7, blood pressure less than 130/80 mmHg, and LDL cholesterol below 100 mg/dL.

D is for diet because weight management is still necessary for long-term health outcomes. It must be remembered that even if a patient's ABC is under control, ageing and weight changes will bring fresh trouble in the future, increasing the risk of complications and the need for medication.

A Better World for People with Diabetes

When I was training to become an endocrinologist forty years ago, the prevalence of diabetes in Delhi was less than

5 per cent. Today, it is around 15 per cent. That means 15 out of 100 adults in Delhi have diabetes, diagnosed or undiagnosed. For people above sixty, the figure is over 35 per cent. Forty years ago, it was unthinkable to see a twenty-year-old with type 2 diabetes. Today, it is a common sight, and we are beginning to see it even among teenagers.

Today, diabetes is all about 'control' – controlling blood sugar levels – but until the mid-1990s, doctors didn't realize the value of controlling blood sugar levels to prevent complications. Shocking as it may seem today, we used to say that a blood glucose reading of 200 mg/dL was acceptable (70–100 mg/dL is ideal for people without diabetes). Nowadays, the usual targets for blood glucose in diabetes patients are between 80 and 120 mg/dL in the fasting state, and below 160–180 mg/dL two hours after a meal. Of course, the targets vary based on age and comorbidities, being tighter for newly diagnosed young individuals and liberal for the elderly. Patients also have a better understanding of the importance of control. If the disease can't be cured, it should at least be minimized.

In the 1980s, glucometers were scarce: there were only two of them in the Endocrinology department at AIIMS! A glucometer was a big black box. Colleagues used to ask us to measure the blood sugar levels of their parents as a favour. Today, technology has made it so easy to measure blood sugar levels that people attach sensors to their arms, tracking sugar levels on their smartphones. The readings can be shared with a relative, doctor or diabetes educator on a real-time basis through apps.

We also have a better understanding of the importance of lipid (cholesterol) and blood pressure control for holistic diabetes management.

In addition to these changes, the medications available to treat diabetes have changed significantly. There used to be only two or three medicines to choose from. It was simple. Within the medical profession, diabetes was quite unglamorous. Endocrinologists in training bothered themselves with more complex medical conditions. After 2000, the exponential growth in diabetes has been unbelievable. Today, many patients think an endocrinologist is essentially a 'diabetes doctor'.

As newer medicines arrived on the scene, they gave doctors better choices to manage diabetes. The drugs available today have made it possible to control blood sugar levels without causing low blood sugar reactions or weight gain, rather inducing weight loss instead. Besides this, some newer anti-diabetes drugs protect organs like the kidney, heart and liver from the effects of the disease. The improvement in diabetes medication options has been as startling as the explosion of diabetes.

A particularly useful advancement was a class of drugs called SGLT2 inhibitors. These throw out excess glucose through the urine. As a result, the excess glucose is not reabsorbed in the body as with some other drugs. Many doctors were sceptical about the potential of these drugs and feared side effects. We were proven wrong. SGLT2 inhibitors proved to be surprisingly effective in lowering sugar levels and are also unexpectedly valuable for preventing kidney disease, a common complication of diabetes. Dapagliflozin and empagliflozin reduced the progression of kidney disease and risk of death by about 30–40 per cent. They also caused some weight loss and helped consistently reduce the risk of heart failure by about 30 per cent. Interestingly, this benefit was seen both in those with and without diabetes.

Another class of drugs, DPP-4 inhibitors, improve the function of natural incretin hormones and have no side effects. But they're not very potent either.

These two types of drugs – SGLT2 and DPP-4 inhibitors – do not cause hypoglycaemia, or low blood sugar, which can be dangerous. Among the older drugs, metformin does not produce low blood sugar. Other diabetes drugs, especially sulphonylureas and insulin, carry this risk. Their glucose-lowering effect is independent of the glucose level, meaning that they will lower your blood sugar levels even if they don't need lowering, even to the point where it can be dangerous.

Some diabetes drugs cause weight gain as a side effect, which raises HbA1c, so you need more medication to keep sugar levels in check. This becomes a vicious cycle. This is true of sulphonylureas, insulin sensitizers like pioglitazone, and insulin itself.

Insulin is the most powerful blood glucose-lowering agent and can rapidly bring down highly elevated blood sugar levels. Some patients may need to take insulin only for a short time, like during an emergency, surgery or pregnancy. Others may need insulin simply because their pancreas has packed up and oral drugs have stopped working. In such cases, insulin is likely to be needed lifelong.

Getting to the Root of the Problem

As we explained in Chapter 1, GLP-1 drugs have been around since 2005, starting with exenatide. But until semaglutide (Ozempic, Wegovy, Rybelsus) came along, the older GLP-1 drugs caused minor weight loss, and the sugar control was not as impressive as with semaglutide or tirzepatide (Mounjaro, Wegovy).

These two new drugs have revolutionized diabetes management. They bring down sugar levels efficiently and quickly without the risk of hypoglycaemia. They also cause significant weight loss, thus addressing the root of the problem. Among those who are overweight and obese but do not have diabetes, the SELECT trial found that weight loss caused by semaglutide (Ozempic, Wegovy) reduced the risk of diabetes by 73 per cent.

Research shows that when an adult male's BMI increases from 18.5 to 35, the risk of diabetes increases from 7 per cent to 70 per cent. Among women, it increases from 12 per cent to 74 per cent. Hence, by addressing the most significant cause of diabetes, GLP-1 drugs have brought about a paradigm shift in diabetes treatment.

With these drugs, we are seeing many more patients send their diabetes into remission and keep it there. Among those with advanced diabetes, I have many patients who find themselves getting rid of their insulin pens and multiple diabetes medications with the aid of new GLP-1 drugs. I often aim to leave patients with only two drugs, GLP-1 and SGLT2 inhibitors, as both of them have extraglycaemic benefits, meaning that they don't only control sugar but also help protect organs, reducing the risk of complications. Combining these two will add many years to patients' lives and ensure a better quality of life.

Except perhaps for DPP-4 inhibitors, all diabetes drugs have side effects. Metformin, the first basic pill given to diabetes patients, causes bloating and gastric side effects such as diarrhoea. SGLT-2 inhibitors cause dehydration, genital infections and sometimes urinary tract infections. Sulphonylureas cause hypoglycaemia. Insulin and insulin sensitizers cause weight gain. Some medications like pioglitazone can even raise the risk of heart failure and osteoporosis.

GLP-1 drugs actually have fewer side effects than most other diabetes drugs, once the initial period of gastrointestinal disturbance has settled down. Just by reducing the need for multiple medicines, other side effects may come down.

Reducing Complications

GLP-1 drugs are also remarkably effective in reducing organ complications, independent of their effect on glucose. Semaglutide (Ozempic, Wegovy) reduced the risk of MACEs (such as heart attacks, brain stroke and cardiovascular death) across a spectrum of people with type 2 diabetes. Overall, semaglutide reduces MACEs in people with type 2 diabetes by about 20 per cent.

In a large study involving more than 3,500 participants, semaglutide 1 mg once a week reduced the risk of kidney failure and death from cardiovascular causes in patients with type 2 diabetes and chronic kidney disease by 24 per cent, over 3.4 years of follow-up. The risk of death was 20 per cent lower in the semaglutide group as compared to the placebo group. In the case of fatty liver disease, semaglutide increased the likelihood of resolution of liver fat, and improvement in steatosis and liver inflammation but did not impact fibrosis.

In one retrospective analysis of more than 72,000 patients, tirzepatide was associated with significantly fewer MACEs outcomes compared to semaglutide in patients with diabetes over a three-year follow-up period. These findings suggest that tirzepatide offers superior cardiovascular protection for primary prevention compared to semaglutide. However, these findings need to be confirmed in further clinical trials.

Another study involving about 2,000 patients followed up for two years, showed that people treated with tirzepatide had fewer renal complications, slower decline in kidney functions and reduced protein leak. Definitive trials in this area are ongoing.

These studies provide evidence that the new GLP-1 drugs have a glucose-independent effect on reducing organ complications among people with diabetes. This finding has profound implications for the role and position of these drugs in diabetes management.

Despite how revolutionary these new drugs are in diabetes management, I barely have any diabetes patients asking me for GLP-1 prescriptions for diabetes management. Usually, I have to push them to try these new drugs.

People with or without diabetes alike want to use these drugs for weight loss. Everyone who is overweight – and, sometimes, those who are not – wants to lose weight for cosmetic purposes. That tells you that people care far more about looking good than their health.

Takeaway

GLP-1 drugs like semaglutide and tirzepatide have ushered in a new era in diabetes management. In many ways, they are ideal anti-diabetes drugs. They control glucose without producing low blood sugar reactions. They produce significant weight loss with all its attendant benefits. Most importantly, they reduce heart, kidney and liver complications caused by the disease, independently of their beneficial effects on blood sugar levels. They have quickly moved up in the hierarchy of diabetes medications.

PATIENT STORY

MADHO GOPAL AGGARWAL, 66

The sight of pakodas, parathas and pickles does not attract me towards them any more. It's as if Mounjaro has put a lock on my head. If anything, I feel irritated seeing these foods. I want them out of my sight. My body and soul reject them. When they are removed from my sight, I feel at peace.

In just four months of Mounjaro, I lost 13 kg. I can barely eat anything – I try to eat half a cup of chana in the morning and I can't even have half of that. I cannot eat much even in the best of breakfast buffets in five-star hotels. I eat roti by dipping it in some milk for dinner. My taste in food has also altered a bit. I have begun eating more fruits, including those I used not to eat much of before I started Mounjaro. My appetite has reduced by three-fourths.

I have had diabetes for 20 years now. Losing 13 kg at the age of sixty-six feels amazing. I feel fitter and look better. Diabetes is the root of many other illnesses, and now I feel happy that I will not be a burden on my family.

At the same time, sometimes I feel a little weak, maybe because I cannot take enough protein due to appetite suppression. As a vegetarian, I try to eat roasted chana with chat masala in the afternoon, followed by some curd rice.

My HbA1c has reduced from 7.9 to 6.5, and I hope it will fall further. Most of my diabetes medicines have been discontinued, though Dr Mithal has continued dapagliflozin. The inconvenience of taking several medicines before and after food is gone. A big relief is that I don't need insulin any more. My cholesterol, sleep apnoea, and a host of other health parameters have improved as well.

I do feel weak and even drowsy sometimes, maybe because I'm barely eating or maybe because I am not consuming enough protein.

I did not have any gastric or intestinal side effects. However, in the two instances where I had poori–aloo for dinner, I had diarrhoea a few hours later. So, I have stopped eating pooris as well.

I wonder how long I will have to be on Mounjaro. I'm sure even better drugs will come out in the future, and I'm willing to try them.

9

The GLP-1 Decade Has Only Just Begun

In medical history, the public launch of semaglutide in 2018 will be considered a watershed moment since it is the first drug to address the meta-disease called obesity in a substantial and impactful manner.

Just as Rome was not built in a day, semaglutide came after a long history of similar drugs based on incretin hormones. The search for more effective anti-diabetes drugs fortuitously led science to the first effective anti-obesity medicine that could produce a weight loss of over 15 per cent.

Intestinal hormones (incretins) are involved in regulating insulin secretion. These are GLP-1 and GIP. Until a few years ago, research focused primarily on developing drugs that would act through the GLP-1 pathway, mimicking the action of native GLP-1. Such drugs have been in use since 2005 – exenatide came first, followed by liraglutide and then dulaglutide. All of these had some weight-loss properties, but except high-dose liraglutide, none made the cut as an anti-obesity drug.

The cupboard of obesity medications was quite bare before semaglutide (Ozempic, Rybelsus, Wegovy) appeared on the scene. With the unprecedented weight loss seen with semaglutide, some thought the peak had been reached with regard to the GLP-1 drugs. However, subsequent development and the commercial launch of a dual receptor agonist, tirzepatide (Mounjaro), which acts via GLP-1 and GIP pathways simultaneously, provided greater benefit, inducing a weight loss of 20 per cent or even more in some cases. Single molecules that are dual and triple receptor agonists are indeed path-breaking discoveries. It's like having the same key unlock two or three different locks. This opens up immense possibilities that could lead to a wide range of hitherto unimagined effects.

Protecting the Liver with Glucagon

We know that tirzepatide (Mounjaro) acts via both GLP-1 and GIP pathways. What about the third hormone, glucagon? Glucagon is secreted from the pancreas, from where it travels to the liver to increase glucose production, and could thus *raise* blood glucose. But glucagon also reduces food intake and increases energy expenditure (a property not found in GLP-1), implying that it could be useful for weight loss. Combining glucagon with GLP-1 actions could improve weight loss while keeping blood glucose under control. Glucagon also results in the improvement of body fat metabolism and promotes liver fatty acid oxidation.

Just as combining GLP-1 and GIP gave us a more potent drug in tirzepatide (Mounjaro), combining glucagon with GLP-1 actions could have its benefits such as better protection for the liver. This could be an excellent option for people with obesity and diabetes who also have fatty liver disease (MASLD).

Such a drug is now in Phase III trial stage. It is called survodutide. It targets GLP-1 and glucagon, leaving out GIP. A key difference between survodutide and the drugs currently available is that it increases energy expenditure and thus fat burning, apart from reducing calorie intake and increasing insulin secretion.

The weight loss achieved with survodutide in trials was 18.7 per cent of total body weight at forty-six weeks. About 40 per cent of participants lost more than 20 per cent of their body weight. For people with diabetes, survodutide twice a week resulted in 9 per cent weight loss, as compared to 5.4 per cent with 1 mg weekly semaglutide. The HbA1c reduction was also superior to semaglutide. The side effects were similar.

The positive results in MASLD are making the US FDA consider fast-tracking the approval of survodutide for this condition. Survodutide has the potential for greater weight loss and greater liver benefit than semaglutide. Further studies will tell us if this potential is realized or not.

Several similar drugs combining GLP-1 with glucagon actions are also in the trial stage.

Triple Action

If targeting two hormones in a single drug is possible and powerful, why not try targeting three?

The quest for further improvements led scientists like Germany's Matthias Tschöp and his collaborators to develop retatrutide, a triple receptor agonist (GLP-1, GIP and glucagon).

Like other GLP-1 drugs, retatrutide is suitable for weekly injection. Clinical results show retatrutide to be better than any GLP-1 drug available so far. Trials showed that full doses of the drug produced weight loss of approximately 25 per cent in forty-eight weeks. Greater weight loss was attained with retatrutide among participants with a BMI of 35 or more. Women lost more weight than men.

Marked improvements in lipid profile (cholesterol) and blood pressure were also observed. There were no 'non-responders'; 100 per cent participants lost at least 5 per cent of their body weight in the same period. In people with diabetes, retatrutide (0.5 to 12 mg) led to a substantial reduction in body weight (16.9 per cent) and HbA1c. The benefits of retatrutide also extended to MASLD as fat content normalized in approximately 90 per cent people receiving the highest doses. As it acts through three pathways, including glucagon, it could be a powerful drug for fatty liver disease.

Something that seemed unimaginable even a few years ago has become a reality: a single molecule that acts via three pathways! It may take a couple of years for retatrutide to become commercially available, provided phase III trials do not show any unexpected adverse effects.

Getting Rid of the Prick

One of the main challenges in GLP-1 drugs is the scarcity and limited efficacy of oral preparations, though semaglutide has partially surmounted that barrier. Oral semaglutide, currently sold under the brand name Rybelsus, while successful in controlling diabetes and showing favourable cardiac outcomes, hasn't been very successful with weight loss. Many companies are working on this because pills are generally more acceptable to patients than injections. If an easily administered oral pill shows data comparable to the injectables, it could have a game-changing impact on obesity management.

Higher doses of oral semaglutide have been tried in an attempt to increase weight loss through the oral route. In a sixty-eight-week phase III trial, oral semaglutide 50 mg resulted in 17.4 per cent weight loss in people with obesity without diabetes, with improvements in multiple cardio-metabolic risk factors. In people with type 2 diabetes, oral semaglutide 50 mg once daily resulted in 9.8 per cent weight loss, as compared to 5.4 per cent with the currently available maximum dose of 14 mg.

I am optimistic about the potential of high-dose oral semaglutide. The benefits (and side effects) depend on how much of the drug reaches the bloodstream. The currently available highest dose, a 14 mg daily pill, achieves blood levels close to those achieved by injecting 1 mg once a week. If 50 mg can achieve levels comparable to those achieved by 2–2.4 mg, there is no reason why it should not be as effective as the injectable version.

A different kind of pill is also in the trial stage. This one, called orforglipron, is not a peptide and, hence, much less sensitive to breakdown in the gut. It can be administered once daily without regard to timing or food intake. Its manufacturer, Eli Lilly, expects to complete phase III trials in 2025, and orforglipron could receive US regulatory approval in 2026.

In trials, orforglipron produced weight loss of 14.7 per cent or 15 kg at thirty-sx weeks, along with a reduction in cardiovascular risk factors. Almost half the people with diabetes achieved 10 per cent or more weight loss after twenty-six weeks of treatment with orforglipron 45 mg.

Greater Weight Loss by Targeting the Amylin Pathway

Amylin is a hormone secreted along with insulin from the pancreas and plays a key role in satiety. It acts on receptors in the brain to reduce food intake and improve glucose metabolism by delaying gastric emptying and inhibiting glucagon secretion. Amylin analogues are drugs that act through the amylin receptor and mimic its action, therefore increasing satiety, reducing food intake and promoting weight loss.

As weight loss with GLP-1 drugs and amylin analogues results from different pathways, it was postulated that a combination of these (GLP-1 and amylin analogues) may produce a synergistic effect, causing more significant weight loss and better sugar control.

Novo Nordisk has developed a new drug, CagriSema, that combines semaglutide with cagrilintide, which is an amylin analogue. The first phase III trial (REDEFINE1) results with CagriSema were released by Novo Nordisk in December 2024. In a sixty-eight-week trial involving 3,417 subjects, CagriSema was compared to the individual components cagrilintide 2.4 mg and semaglutide 2.4 mg administered weekly. The mean baseline body weight was 106.9 kg. People treated with CagriSema achieved a superior weight loss of 22.7 per cent after sixty-eight weeks compared to 11.8 per cent with cagrilintide 2.4 mg and 16.1 per cent with semaglutide 2.4 mg.

However, gastrointestinal adverse effects with CagriSema were greater than with semaglutide or cagrilintide monotherapy, though they did not lead to higher discontinuation rates.

Meanwhile, Novo Nordisk has also developed a single molecule called amycretin that acts via both the GLP-1 and amylin pathways. This has both oral and injectable versions. In early trials, at twelve weeks, patients with obesity taking amycretin lost an average of more than 10 per cent of their body weight.

In January 2025, topline results from an early-phase clinical trial with the weekly injectable amycretin were announced by the company. One-hundred-twenty-five people with a mean baseline weight of 92.7 kg were treated for thirty-six weeks. People treated with the maximal doses (20 mg) lost 22 per cent weight.

Maintaining Weight Loss

Amgen, a biotechnology company, has adopted a unique approach in developing a drug called MariTide. It is an antibody peptide conjugate, meaning it combines two molecules with very different structures. MariTide activates GLP-1 receptors while – hold your breath – *reducing* GIP activity. Such is the complexity of GLP-1 biology! The biggest advantage of this drug is that it is a monthly injection, not weekly.

Early trial data was released in November 2024. In people with obesity or overweight without diabetes, MariTide demonstrated up to 20 per cent average weight loss at week 52, without a weight-loss plateau, indicating the potential for further weight loss beyond fifty-two weeks.

In people with type 2 diabetes, who typically lose less weight on GLP-1 therapies, MariTide achieved up to 17 per cent average weight loss, also without a weight-loss plateau, and lowered their average HbA1c by up to 2.2 percentage points at week 52. The potential for continued weight loss beyond fifty-two weeks makes this drug an exciting prospect.

MariTide also demonstrated a robust reduction of cardio-metabolic parameters, including blood pressure and triglycerides. It has been reported that, unlike other treatments, MariTide has shown the ability to *maintain* weight loss for several months after the last dose. If proven in further studies, this might be a huge advantage since one of the significant challenges with semaglutide or tirzepatide is the rapid weight gain that can occur upon discontinuation of the drug.

Build Muscle While Losing Weight

The biggest challenge with rapid weight loss, with or without medication, is that some muscle loss invariably accompanies the fat loss. Typically, 20–30 per cent of the weight lost is muscle mass. Ensuring adequate protein intake and resistance training is the only way to minimize the loss. If someone goes through a weight loss-and-regain cycle repeatedly, they will be left with progressively less muscle and greater fat mass. Attempts are being made to develop medications that preserve or even promote muscle mass, while simultaneously inducing fat loss.

In a small, early-phase trial involving overweight or obese patients (BMI 28–40) with type 2 diabetes, those who received the monoclonal antibody bimagrumab had a significantly larger decrease in total body fat mass and HbA1c, and an increase in lean mass compared to patients who received placebo.

Bimagrumab is given as a monthly intravenous infusion, which involves hospital daycare. It blocks activin type II receptors and stimulates skeletal muscle growth.

The rise in muscle mass accompanied by fat loss is quite unique. It seems unlikely, though, that bimagrumab alone will be as effective as GLP-1 drugs in promoting weight loss. Eli Lilly is currently running a trial combining bimagrumab with tirzepatide in the hope of producing significant weight loss and improving muscle mass at the same time.

The hormone testosterone plays an important role in building and preserving muscle. A category of drugs in trial stages known as SARMs, or selective androgen receptor modulators, mimics the anabolic (muscle-building) effects of the male hormone testosterone but with reduced androgenic (masculinizing) properties. One such drug being tried is enobosarm, a daily pill. Enobosarm treatment in cancer leads to dose-dependent increases in muscle mass with improvements in physical function and significant reductions in fat mass. The patient data generated from enobosarm clinical trials in elderly patients and patients with cancer-induced appetite suppression provide a strong clinical rationale that enobosarm, in combination with a GLP-1 drug, could reduce body fat while preserving muscle mass.

Novo Nordisk conducted an early-phase study using enobosarm 3 mg and 6 mg in 168 patients greater than 60 years of age receiving semaglutide. The topline results declared in January 2025 showed that, on average, patients on enobosarm lost 71 per cent less lean mass and 27 per cent more fat mass compared to patients receiving semaglutide alone. The total body weight lost was the same in both groups. Enobosarm reduced the proportion of patients who lost clinically significant physical function compared to subjects receiving semaglutide alone.

A Cupboard Full of Options

The field of obesity research is abuzz with excitement, with many new drugs in the pipeline. The speed of research and discovery in obesity treatment is breathtaking. In 2024 and 2025, every month has seen a major new advance in obesity treatment. Around a hundred different drugs are reportedly in trial stage worldwide.

Some challenges remain. The gastrointestinal side effects seem to be part and parcel of GLP-1 drugs, and little improvement has taken place in this direction. They continue to be bothersome for some people and are the chief reason for discontinuing the drugs. Slow-dose titration remains the best way to circumvent these effects.

Most GLP-1 drugs are injectables. While oral drugs have met with some success, the dose of medication needed is much higher and could potentially be challenging to maintain supplies.

The high cost of these drugs makes them out of reach for large segments of the Indian population. It is hoped that the innovator companies will rationalize prices as sales increase. Besides, the expiry of patents of some drugs will enable generic drug manufacturers to manufacture and supply these drugs at much lower, competitive prices.

A wide variety of drug choices is likely to be available. Ultimately, we will have several drugs, each with its unique properties. Some may be oral, others may be muscle-preserving, while yet another may work specifically for the liver. Some of these molecules will fall by the wayside, some will carve a niche position for themselves, and some will be blockbusters.

The efficacy of semaglutide (Ozempic, Wegovy) and tripeptide (Mounjaro, Zepbound) has raised the bar for new molecules. Three years ago, a drug that produced 20 per cent weight loss would have been considered sensational. Now, 20 per cent weight loss with a new drug is considered disappointing and may even cause the company's share prices to fall. Eli Lilly's triple receptor agonist retatrutide has led the way in potency, with almost 25 per cent weight loss seen in those without diabetes.

Buckle up! We are in for exciting times in our battle against the bulge.

Takeaway

The current GLP-1 drugs are likely to be succeeded by many better variants that are likely to produce greater weight loss, minimize muscle loss, be easier to take, and may be customized for specific comorbidities like fatty liver disease – hopefully with fewer side effects.

PATIENT STORY

ARUN SINGH, 52*

I started with Ozempic and recently switched to Mounjaro. Before starting Ozempic, my HbA1C was 9. The drugs have been very good in controlling my sugar, bringing my HbA1C to 6.2. In fact, at one point, it had come down to 5.4, but perhaps I ate too many sweets in the festive season.

I lost almost no weight on Ozempic, but on Mounjaro, I have lost 5–6 kg. These drugs gave me constipation for the first time in my life. I hope in the future there will be better ones that will not give me constipation.

Yet I have no complaints. When your sugar is at an HbA1C of 9, you always feel tired, anxious and irritable. With sugar control, I'm now in a happy space. I take only one more medicine to control my sugar.

The appetite control with Mounjaro ensures that even if I eat sweets, it is just one piece. The mind rejects the idea of a second serving. I eat breakfast at 9 a.m. and dinner at 8 p.m., so I'm effectively intermittent fasting for twelve–fourteen hours.

---

*Name changed to protect privacy.

I used to play sports, but obesity and diabetes are in my DNA. There's a family history. At one point, I reached 140 kg. I made a lot of effort to come down to 95 kg but gained a lot of weight again. At fifty-two, I'm not able to push my body to exercise the way I could at forty. With Mounjaro, my sugar control and some weight loss have both happened without me having to push myself.

My wife also started with Ozempic and switched to Mounjaro. Her experience has been completely the opposite. Her sugar control on Ozempic was phenomenal, and she has lost a lot of weight. She hasn't lost much incremental weight on Mounjaro.

Bibliography

Abbass, Nadia J, Raya Nahlawi, Jacqueline K Shaia, Kevin C Allan, David C Kaelber, Katherine E Talcott, and Rishi P Singh. 2025. The Effect of Semaglutide and GLP-1 RAs on Risk of Non-Arteritic Anterior Ischemic Optic Neuropathy. *American Journal of Ophthalmology*, February.

Abushamat LA, Shah PA, Eckel RH, Harrison SA, Barb D. The emerging role of glucagon-like peptide-1 receptor agonists for the treatment of metabolic dysfunction-associated steatohepatitis. Clin Gastroenterol Hepatol, 22:1565–74, 2024.

Anjana RM, Unnikrishnan R, Deepa M, et al. Metabolic non-communicable disease health report of India: the ICMR-INDIAB national cross-sectional study (ICMR-INDIAB-17). Lancet Diabetes Endocrinol, 11:474–89, 2023.

'As Many as 1 in 5 People Won't Lose Weight with Glp-1 Drugs, Experts Say.' 2024. Cbsnews.com. CBS News. November 25, 2024. https://www.cbsnews.com/news/1-in-5-people-wont-lose-weight-glp-1-drugs-experts/.

Austregésilo de Athayde De Hollanda Morais B, Martins Prizão V, de Moura de Souza M, et al. The efficacy and safety of GLP-1 agonists in PCOS women living with obesity in promoting weight loss and hormonal regulation: A meta-analysis of randomized controlled trials. J Diabetes Complications, 38:108834, 2024.

Ayoub M, Chela H, Amin N, et al. Pancreatitis risk associated with GLP-1 receptor agonists, considered as a single class, in a comorbidity-free subgroup of type 2 diabetes patients in the United States: A propensity score-matched analysis. **J Clin Med**, 14:944, 2025.

Bawa T, Dhingra V, Malhotra N, Wasir JS, Mithal A. Clinical experience with exenatide in obese North Indian patients with type 2 diabetes mellitus. Indian J Endocrinol Metab, 17:91–4, 2013.

Bellentani S, Saccoccio G, Masutti F, et al. Prevalence of and risk factors for hepatic steatosis in Northern Italy. Ann Intern Med, 132:112–17, 2000.

Abate, Carolyn. 2016. 'Body Shaming on Social Media.' Healthline. 2016. https://www.healthline.com/health-news/body-shaming-in-social-media.

Bosch C, Carriazo S, Soler MJ, Ortiz A, Fernandez-Fernandez B. Tirzepatide and prevention of chronic kidney disease. Clin Kidney J, 16:797–808, 2023.

Cervantes M, Miles B, Mehta A. Comparison of cardiovascular outcomes in patients with diabetes treated with tirzepatide versus semaglutide: a multi-institutional analysis. Eur Heart J, 45:ehae666.2907, 2024.

Chavda VP, Balar PC, Vaghela DA, Dodiya P. Unlocking longevity with GLP-1: A key to turn back the clock? Maturitas, 186:108028, 2024.

Dao K, Shechtman S, Weber-Schoendorfer C, et al. Use of GLP1 receptor agonists in early pregnancy and reproductive safety: a multicentre, observational, prospective cohort study based on the databases of six Teratology Information Services. BMJ Open, 14:e083550, 2024.

de Lemos JA, Linetzky B, le Roux CW, et al. Deanfield J, Verma S, Scirica BM, et al. Semaglutide and cardiovascular outcomes in patients with obesity and prevalent heart failure: A prespecified analysis of the SELECT trial. Lancet, 404:773–86, 2024.

Donnelly, Laura. 2022. Extra Inches on the Waistline 'Biggest Risk for Heart Disease.' The Telegraph. August 28, 2022. https://www.telegraph.co.uk/news/2022/08/28/extra-inches-waistline-biggest-risk-heart-disease/?ICID=continue_without_subscribing_reg_first.

Drucker DJ, Habener JF, Holst JJ. Discovery, characterization, and clinical development of the glucagon-like peptides. J Clin Invest, 127:4217–27, 2017.

Dutta A, Mahendru S, Sharma R, Mithal A. Effectiveness of oral semaglutide in management of type 2 diabetes: A real-world study from India. Indian J Endocrinol Metab, 28:653–8, 2024.

Eknoyan G. A history of obesity, or how what was good became ugly and then bad. Adv Chronic Kidney Dis, 13:421–7, 2006.

'Exendin-4: From Lizard to Laboratory...And Beyond.' 2012. National Institute on Aging. July 11, 2012. https://www.nia.nih.gov/news/exendin-4-lizard-laboratory-and-beyond.

Foer D, Strasser ZH, Cui J, et al. Association of GLP-1 receptor agonists with chronic obstructive pulmonary disease exacerbations among patients with type 2 diabetes. Am J Respir Crit Care Med, 208:1088–100, 2023.

Friedman JM. The discovery and development of GLP-1 based drugs that have revolutionized the treatment of obesity. Proc Natl Acad Sci U.S.A., 121:e2415550121, 2024.

GBD 2021 Adult BMI Collaborators. Global, regional, and national prevalence of adult overweight and obesity, 1990–2021, with forecasts to 2050: a forecasting study for the Global Burden of Disease Study 2021. Lancet, 405:813–38, 2025.

Ghusn W, Hurtado MD. Glucagon-like receptor-1 agonists for obesity: Weight loss outcomes, tolerability, side effects, and risks. Obes Pillars, 12:100127, 2024.

GLP-1 receptor agonists: new treatment frontiers. Nat Mental Health 3, 267–8, 2025.

GLP-1 receptor agonists: reminder of the potential side effects and to be aware of the potential for misuse. https://www.gov.uk/drug-safety-update/glp-1-receptor-agonists-reminder-of-the-potential-side-effects-and-to-be-aware-of-the-potential-for-misuse, 2024.

GLP-1s like Ozempic are among the most important drug breakthroughs ever, https://www.economist.com/briefing/2024/10/24/glp-1s-like-ozempic-are-among-the-most-important-drug-breakthroughs-ever, 2024.

Guglielmi G. The weight-loss drugs being tested in 2025: Will they beat Ozempic? Nature, 638:591–2, 2025.

Hall, Kevin D., and Scott Kahan. 2018. Maintenance of Lost Weight and Long-Term Management of Obesity. *Medical Clinics of North America* 102 (1): 183–97.

Bibliography

Harris, Emily. 2024. Poll: Roughly 12% of US Adults Have Used a GLP-1 Drug, Even If Unaffordable. *JAMA* 332 (1): 8–8.

Hathaway JT, Shah MP, Hathaway DB, et al. Risk of nonarteritic anterior ischemic optic neuropathy in patients prescribed semaglutide. JAMA Ophthalmol, 142:732–9, 2024.

Hendershot CS, Bremmer MP, Paladino MB, et al. Once-weekly semaglutide in adults with alcohol use disorder: A randomized clinical trial. JAMA Psychiatry, 2025.

Her work paved the way for blockbuster obesity drugs. Now, she's fighting for recognition. https://www.science.org/content/article/her-work-paved-way-blockbuster-obesity-drugs-now-she-s-fighting-recognition, 2023.

Hinte, Laura C., Daniel Castellano-Castillo, Adhideb Ghosh, Kate Melrose, Emanuel Gasser, Falko Noé, Lucas Massier, et al. 2024. Adipose Tissue Retains an Epigenetic Memory of Obesity after Weight Loss. *Nature*, November.

Husain M, Bain SC, Jeppesen OK, et al. Semaglutide (SUSTAIN and PIONEER) reduces cardiovascular events in type 2 diabetes across varying cardiovascular risk. Diabetes Obes Metab, 22:442–51, 2020.

Jackson SE, Beeken RJ, Wardle J. Perceived weight discrimination and changes in weight, waist circumference, and weight status. Obesity (Silver Spring), 22:2485–8, 2014.

Jastreboff AM, Kaplan LM, Frías JP, et al. Triple-hormone-receptor agonist retatrutide for obesity – A phase 2 trial. N Engl J Med, 389:514–26, 2023.

Jensterle M, Rizzo M, Haluzík M, Janež A. Efficacy of GLP-1 RA approved for weight management in patients with or without diabetes: A narrative review. Adv Ther, 39:2452–67, 2022.

Bibliography

Jiang F, Li G, Ji W, et al. Obesity is associated with decreased gray matter volume in children: a longitudinal study. Cerebral Cortex, 33:3674–82, 2023.

Kahn, Steven E, John E Deanfield, Ole Kleist Jeppesen, Scott S Emerson, Trine Welløv Boesgaard, Helen M Colhoun, Robert F Kushner, et al. Effect of Semaglutide on Regression and Progression of Glycemia in People with Overweight or Obesity but without Diabetes in the SELECT Trial. *Diabetes Care*, June. 2024.

Kalra S, Kapoor N, Verma M, Shaikh S, Das S, Jacob J, Sahay R. Defining and diagnosing obesity in India: A call for advocacy and action. J Obes, 1:4178121, 2023.

Kanbour S, Ageeb RA, Malik RA, Abu-Raddad LJ. Impact of bodyweight loss on type 2 diabetes remission: a systematic review and meta-regression analysis of randomised controlled trials. Lancet Diabetes Endocrinol, 13:294–306, 2025.

Karamanou M, Protogerou A, Tsoucalas G, Androutsos G, Poulakou-Rebelakou E. Milestones in the history of diabetes mellitus: The main contributors. World J Diabetes, 7:1–7, 2016.

Kaur P, Mahendru S, Mithal A. Long-term efficacy of liraglutide in Indian patients with type 2 diabetes in a real-world setting. Indian J Endocrinol Metab, 20:595–9, 2016.

Kaur P, Mishra SK, Mithal A, Saxena M, Makkar A, Sharma P. Clinical experience with liraglutide in 196 patients with type 2 diabetes from a tertiary care centre in India. Indian J Endocrinol Metab, 18:77–82, 2014.

Kernan WN, Inzucchi SE, Sawan C, Macko RF, Furie KL. Obesity: A stubbornly obvious target for stroke prevention. Stroke, 44:278–86, 2013.

Kiliaan AJ, Arnoldussen IA, Gustafson DR. Adipokines: A link between obesity and dementia? Lancet Neurol,13:913–23, 2014.

Kolata, Gina. 2025. The Physicians Really Are Healing Themselves, with Ozempic. *The New York Times*, February 10, 2025. https://www.nytimes.com/2025/02/10/health/doctors-ozempic-weight-loss.html.

Kreiner FF, von Scholten BJ, Kurtzhals P, Gough SCL. Glucagon-like peptide-1 receptor agonists to expand the healthy lifespan: Current and future potentials. Aging Cell, 22:e13818, 2023.

Kuchay MS, Krishan S, Mishra SK, et al. Effect of dulaglutide on liver fat in patients with type 2 diabetes and NAFLD: Randomised controlled trial (D-LIFT trial). Diabetologia, 63:2434–45, 2020.

Kurth T, Gaziano JM, Berger K, et al. Body mass index and the risk of stroke in men. Arch Intern Med, 162:2557–62, 2002.

Lopez-Jimenez F, Almahmeed W, Bays H, et al. Obesity and cardiovascular disease: Mechanistic insights and management strategies. A joint position paper by the World Heart Federation and World Obesity Federation. Eur J Prev Cardiol, 29:2218–23, 2022.

Sri Ventakta, Nitin Kapoor, Sambit Das, Nishant Raizada, Sanjay Kalra. 'ESI Clinical Practice Guidelines for the Evaluation and Management of Obesity In India'. *Indian Journal of Endocrinology and Metabolism*. 2022 July–August. 26(4):295-318. doi: 10.4103/2230-8210.356236.

Mandal S, Jaganathan S, Kondal D, et al. PM2.5 exposure, glycemic markers and incidence of type 2 diabetes in two large Indian cities: BMJ Open Diabetes ResCare, 11:e003333, 2023.

Matthews A, Herrett E, Gasparrini A, et al. Impact of statin related media coverage on use of statins: interrupted time series analysis with UK primary care data BMJ, 353:i3283, 2016.

McCoy RG, Herrin J, Swarna KS, et al. Effectiveness of glucose-lowering medications on cardiovascular outcomes in patients with type 2 diabetes at moderate cardiovascular risk. Nat Cardiovasc Res, 3:431–40, 2024.

Melson E, Ashraf U, Papamargaritis D. What is the pipeline for future medications for obesity? Int J Obes (Lond), 2024.

Morinaga, Hironobu, Yasuaki Mohri, Marina Grachtchouk, Kyosuke Asakawa, Hiroyuki Matsumura, Motohiko Oshima, Naoya Takayama, et al. 2021. Obesity Accelerates Hair Thinning by Stem Cell-Centric Converging Mechanism. *Nature* 595 (7866): 266–71.

Narayan, K.M.V., J. P. Boyle, T. J. Thompson, E. W. Gregg, and D. F. Williamson. 2007. Effect of BMI on Lifetime Risk for Diabetes in the U.S. *Diabetes Care* 30 (6): 1562–66.

Nauck MA, Quast DR, Wefers J, Pfeiffer AFH. The evolving story of incretins (GIP and GLP-1) in metabolic and cardiovascular disease: A pathophysiological update. Diabetes Obes Metab, 23:5–29, 2021.

Nielsen SF, Nordestgaard BG. Negative statin-related news stories decrease statin persistence and increase myocardial infarction and cardiovascular mortality: a nationwide prospective cohort study. Eur Heart J, 37:908–16, 2016.

Nørgaard CH, Friedrich S, Hansen CT, et al. Treatment with

glucagon-like peptide-1 receptor agonists and incidence of dementia: Data from pooled double-blind randomized controlled trials and nationwide disease and prescription registers. Alzheimers Dement (N Y), 8:e12268, 2022.

Obesity and overweight, https://www.who.int/news-room/fact-sheets/detail/obesity-and-overweight, 2024.

Osler, Sir William. The Principles and Practice of Medicine: Designed for the Use of Practitioners and Students of Medicine, D. Appleton and Company, 1892.

Overview: Diabetes medicines: GLP-1 agonists, https://www.guysandstthomas.nhs.uk/health-information/diabetes-medicines-glp-1-agonists, 2022.

Perkovic, Vlado. 2024. Effects of Semaglutide on Chronic Kidney Disease in Patients with type 2 Diabetes. *New England Journal of Medicine/the New England Journal of Medicine* 391 (2).

Pratley, Richard E, Vanita R Aroda, Ildiko Lingvay, Jörg Lüdemann, Camilla Andreassen, Andrea Navarria, and Adie Viljoen. 2018. Semaglutide versus Dulaglutide Once Weekly in Patients with type 2 Diabetes (Sustain 7): A Randomised, Open-Label, Phase 3B Trial. *The Lancet Diabetes & Endocrinology* 6 (4): 275–86.

Rajagopalan, Sanjay, Robert D Brook, Pedro, Brendan Bourges-Sevenier, Philip Landrigan, Mark J Nieuwenhuijsen, Thomas Munzel, Salil V Deo, and Sadeer Al-Kindi. 2024. Air Pollution Exposure and Cardiometabolic Risk. *The Lancet Diabetes & Endocrinology*, February.

Rivera FB, Cruz LLA, Magalong JV, et al. Cardiovascular and renal outcomes of glucagon-like peptide 1 receptor agonists among patients with and without type 2 diabetes mellitus: A meta-analysis of randomized placebo-controlled trials. Am J Prev Cardiol, 18:100679, 2024.

Ryan DH, Lingvay I, Deanfield J, et al. Long-term weight loss effects of semaglutide in obesity without diabetes in the SELECT trial. Nat Med, 30:2049–57,2024.

Shenker MN, Shalitin S. Use of GLP-1 receptor agonists for the management of type 1 diabetes: A pediatric perspective. *Horm Res Paediatr,* 1–20, 2024.

Singh, Romil, Sawai Singh Rathore, Hira Khan, Smruti Karale, Yogesh Chawla, Kinza Iqbal, Abhishek Bhurwal, et al. 2022. Association of Obesity with COVID-19 Severity and Mortality: An Updated Systemic Review, Meta-Analysis, and Meta-Regression. *Frontiers in Endocrinology* 13 (June).

Tirzepatide reduces 24-hour ambulatory blood pressure in adults with body mass index ≥27 kg/m^2: SURMOUNT-1 Ambulatory Blood Pressure Monitoring Substudy. Hypertension, 81:e41–3, 2024.

Use of semaglutide and risk of non-arteritic anterior ischemic optic neuropathy: A Danish–Norwegian cohort study. medRxiv. Published online doi: 10.1101/2024.12.09.24318574 202.

Von Behren J, Lipsett M, Horn-Ross PL, et al. Obesity, waist size and prevalence of current asthma in the California Teachers Study cohort. Thorax, 64:889–93, 2009.

Wang, Lindsey, Rong Xu, David C Kaelber, and Nathan A Berger. 2024. Glucagon-like Peptide 1 Receptor Agonists and 13 Obesity-Associated Cancers in Patients with type 2 Diabetes. *JAMA Network Open* 7 (7): e2421305–5.

Wang L, Wang Q, Li L, Kaelber DC, Xu R. Glucagon-like

peptide-1 receptor agonists and pancreatic cancer risk: target trial emulation using real-world data. J Natl Cancer Inst, 117:476–85, 2025.

Wasir JS, Mithal A, Agarwal P, Mittal A. Once weekly dulaglutide therapy in type 2 diabetic subjects, real-world evidence from a tertiary care diabetes centre in India. Indian J Endocrinol Metab, 22:728–34, 2018.

Wharton S, Calanna S, Davies M, et al. Gastrointestinal tolerability of once-weekly semaglutide 2.4 mg in adults with overweight or obesity, and the relationship between gastrointestinal adverse events and weight loss. Diabetes Obes Metab, 24:94–105, 2022.

Yao H, Zhang A, Li D, et al. Comparative effectiveness of GLP-1 receptor agonists on glycaemic control, body weight, and lipid profile for type 2 diabetes: systematic review and network meta-analysis. BMJ, 384:e076410, 2024.

Yashi K, Daley SF. Obesity and type 2 diabetes. StatPearls Publishing, Treasure Island, USA, 2023.

Acknowledgements

This book was a fast-track project, made possible by the unwavering and unstinted cooperation of my wife Ranjana, and our children Kreeti, Varun, Sonika and Vibhav.

Even Snoopy understood and left me alone, for which I am highly thankful.

I could not have found a better collaborator than Shivam, who now knows more about weight loss medications than most doctors. Chiki kept a close eye on the progress and egged us on, ensuring we finished in time. Many thanks to both of them.

A Note on the Authors

Dr Ambrish Mithal is the chairman and head of endocrinology and diabetes at Max Healthcare. He is a recipient of numerous awards which include the Padma Bhushan and the Dr B.C. Roy Award from the President of India, both in 2015. He is also the first and only Indian to receive the Laureate Award for International Excellence in Endocrinology by the Endocrine Society (US) in 2021.

Shivam Vij is a writer based in Delhi. He has been trying to lose weight for many years.